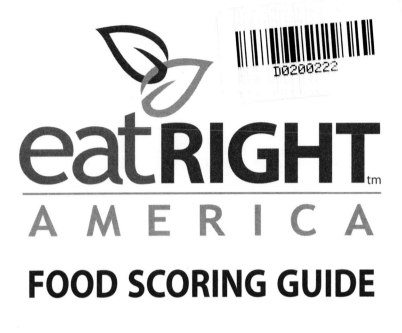

FOOD SCORING GUIDE

JOEL FUHRMAN, M.D.

Nutritional Excellence, LLC

For information, contact:
Nutritional Excellence, LLC
(877) 372-4872
www.EatRightAmerica.com

Printed in the United States of America

ISBN: 0-974463-38-8
ISBN-13: 978-0974463-38-4

Library of Congress Control Number: 2007931556

Publisher's Note:
Keep in mind that results vary from person to person.
Some people have a medical history and/or condition
that may warrant individualized recommendation and, in
some cases, drugs and even surgery. Do not start, stop, or
change medication without professional medical advice,
and do not change your diet if you are ill or on medication,
except under the supervision of a competent physician.
Neither this, nor any other book, is intended to take the
place of personalized medical care or treatment.

For reasons of privacy, the names of patients have been
changed.

Book design: Lennon Media, Inc.
Cover design: Creative Syndicate, Inc.

*Dedicated to Americans who are taking steps
to improve our nation's health*

Contents

Foreword ix

Introduction 1

1. America's Health Crisis and *You* 3
2. Dramatic Results Without Drugs 23
3. Measuring Nutrient Density 41
4. You Are *What* You Eat! 55
5. High-Nutrient Recipes........................ 63
6. Your Commitment to Health 79
7. Dr. Fuhrman's Top 30 Super Foods 83
8. Nutrient Density Scores....................... 85

References....................................... 127
A Message from the Publisher 131
About the Author 132

Foreword

Modern America is in the midst of an all-you-can-eat food fest that has us literally bursting at the seams. Clearly, we eat too much and too often, but we also eat all the wrong foods. The standard American diet now consists of 52% processed foods and 41% meats and dairy products. The most healthful foods—fruits and vegetables—make up only 7% of our national diet.

Eating the wrong foods leads us to consume far too many calories. The average American consumes 3600 calories per day, nearly twice as many as we need. However, because all of these excess calories come from low-nutrient foods, most Americans are significantly undernourished. The Center for Disease Control (CDC) estimates that an astonishing 95% of all Americans fail to get the minimum daily requirement of nutrients. When you factor in the sedentary lifestyle most Americans have adopted (three out of ten American adults did not exercise even *once* last year), you have the perfect recipe for the obesity and chronic illness epidemics that are sweeping the nation.

The World Health Organization now ranks the United States as the fattest nation on earth—including children. The CDC now estimates that one-half of all children will be overweight by 2010, and that for the first time in our nation's history, the current generation of children will not live as long as their parents. In spite of our spending more on healthcare than any other nation, America's children are developing "adult" chronic illnesses such as heart disease, asthma, allergies, hypertension, type 2 diabetes, and even some cancers at much earlier ages.

I have studied epidemiology for more than 30 years, and one thing has become crystal clear—nutrition is powerful medicine. We don't have to be a sickly nation with illnesses and medical costs spiraling out of control. But to restore health to America, we need to make fundamental changes in our eating habits, and we need to make them fast.

Fortunately, you don't need to wait until everybody else changes; you can make the vitally necessary changes today. I urge you to adopt the eating principles described in this book. Dr. Fuhrman is one of the world's authorities on the effects of optimal nutrition on health. He has spent the past 20 years analyzing over 20,000 scientific studies and devising dietary programs that take advantage of his findings. I have witnessed firsthand the results of his remarkable efforts. In most cases, diseases such as heart disease, diabetes, high blood pressure, and obesity simply disappear as a result of patients adopting the dietary principles described in this book.

Dr. Fuhrman has put his scientific knowledge into action in the kitchen. He has tested his methods with patients for more than 15 years and has convinced me and many of my colleagues that a diet of nutrient-rich foods can prevent and cure obesity and most of America's health problems. In fact, a study on Dr. Fuhrman's approach, done in association with Barbara Sarter, Ph.D., of the University of Southern California and Dr. T. Colin Campbell, Ph.D., of Cornell University found that the people who followed his dietary recommendations lost more weight *than in any other study in medical history.* They also kept the weight off through the two-year follow-up.

To take advantage of Dr. Fuhrman's high-nutrient diet, you need to increase your intake of high-nutrient foods and decrease your intake of low-nutrient foods. But how do you know which ones are which? One of the most powerful and revealing elements of Dr. Fuhrman's work is his food rating system—Aggregate Nutrient Density Index (ANDI). ANDI is presented in this book to help you understand the differences between high-nutrient foods and those lacking in important nutrients. This food rating system also shows you caloric density, which helps you avoid high-calorie, low-nutrient foods. It will change the way you think about foods.

If you have tried to lose weight but failed using traditional or fad diets, this book is for you. Follow Dr. Fuhrman's advice, and you will lose weight and keep it off. If you are tired of taking cholesterol-lowering medications, blood pressure medications, or other prescriptions that do nothing but treat symptoms without addressing the underlying cause of your ailment, this book is for you. You will be amazed at what optimal nutrition can do for you. If you are raising a family, this book offers tremendous benefits for you and your children. Not only will you and your family benefit greatly through enhanced health and longevity, your medical bills will go down as well.

In this book (and more extensively in his comprehensive two-book set, *Eat For Health)*, Dr. Fuhrman takes the best of the world's nutritional research, makes it understandable, and shows you how to put it to work in your everyday life. Now you can control your weight and health destiny like never before. The information in this book may save your life.

A. William Menzin, M.D., M.Sc., M.P.H.
Clinical Psychiatry, Nutritional Epidemiology,
and International Health
Harvard Medical School (1974-2006)

Introduction

No one wants to have a heart attack, suffer a debilitating stroke, or develop cancer. But lots of people die from these conditions every day...*unnecessarily*.

Nutritional science has made dramatic advances in recent years. The overwhelming accumulation of scientific knowledge points to a dramatic conclusion—*the majority of diseases plaguing Americans are preventable*. Using the information gleaned from scientific studies, it is now possible to formulate a few simple diet and lifestyle principles that can save you years of suffering and premature death. You have an unprecedented opportunity in human history to live healthier and longer than ever before.

But living healthier and longer comes at a price.

How much would it be worth to you for a guarantee that you would never have a heart attack or a stroke? What would it be worth to you to see your children and grandchildren grow healthfully and happily? What would you be willing to pay for the assurance that you would not leave your spouse or your children all alone?

Fortunately, the expenditure is infinitely affordable—little more than the effort needed to establish new, more healthful eating habits.

Everything in this book is carefully referenced to recent scientific studies. Still, the facts and guidelines contained herein will astound most physicians. Although the research is readily available for all to see, most physicians still have no idea that food can be your most powerful artillery in the fight against the major illnesses that plague Americans.

Chapter One

America's Health Crisis and *You*

A mericans are digging their graves with their knives and forks. Most people in America are overweight, and about half of us are taking drugs for chronic illnesses. Last year alone, 400,000 Americans died from obesity and the weight-related chronic illnesses that develop as a result of being overweight. The poor diet that Americans eat also has resulted in an epidemic of heart attacks and cancer never before seen in human history. We literally are eating ourselves to death.

The ever increasing waistline of America is not merely a cosmetic issue. This march toward national obesity is taking a dramatic toll on our health and the economy, and is causing medical and financial tragedies for more and more families. At present, two-thirds (67%) of American adults, and nearly one-third (31%) of our children, are overweight or obese. Over the past thirty years, the average weight of an

3

American male has increased 27 pounds (from 164 pounds to 191 pounds). Childhood obesity has tripled over the past twenty years. Because of America's eating habits, the U.S. Center for Disease Control (CDC) predicts that the current generation of children will be the first in our nation's history to live shorter lives than their parents.

Health Complications of Obesity

- *Increased overall mortality*
- *Adult onset diabetes*
- *Hypertension*
- *Degenerative arthritis*
- *Coronary artery disease*
- *Obstructive sleep apnea*
- *Gallstones*
- *Fatty infiltration of liver*
- *Restrictive lung disease*
- *Cancer*

Overweight individuals are more likely to die from all causes, including heart disease and cancer.

Food, food everywhere

Food is available and eaten in so many places—the car, the office, the TV room, the movies, the ball game, the gas station...virtually everywhere—that America is fast becoming an all-you-can-eat buffet. And we are almost always selecting the wrong foods.

Americans have access to a greater abundance of affordable high-nutrient, low-calorie fruits and vegetables than any other people on the face of the earth. But a shocking 93% of the typical American diet consists of low-nutrient, high-calorie processed foods, animal foods, and dairy products, and only 7% of the calories we consume come from healthful fruits and vegetables. Sweets, desserts, and soft drinks now comprise 25% of all calories consumed in America.

Composition of the American Diet

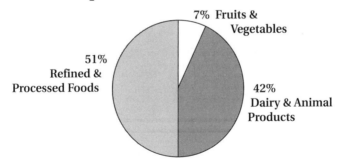

7% Fruits & Vegetables

51% Refined & Processed Foods

42% Dairy & Animal Products

American diet designed for disease

The U.S. Surgeon General classifies overweight and obesity as two stages of a single disease and has called our current eating habits a greater threat to our nation's health and economy than terrorism or bird flu. The Surgeon General's assessment of America's eating habits (which in all likelihood means *your* eating habits) is critically important because bad eating habits lead to bigger problems than just larger dress sizes. They are causing the record-high rates of heart disease, strokes, diabetes, and cancer that are plaguing the country. People of all weights, shapes, and sizes are dying needlessly from nutritional ignorance.

Broken hearts

We are losing the war against heart disease. One hundred years ago, heart disease only affected 5% of the population. Today, it affects almost all Americans as cardiovascular-related deaths have climbed to over 50%. Heart disease (cardiovascular disease) kills more people than the next four leading causes of death *combined*. Modern medical techniques and drugs cannot win this war because the true cause of disease is overlooked. Heart disease is caused by inadequate nutrition.

Impact of heart disease on America
- *40% of all Americans die of heart attacks.*
- *58% of deaths are related to cardiovascular disease.*
- *10% die of strokes.*

The tragedy of this is enormous. More than 1.3 million Americans will suffer a heart attack this year, and when you consider that nobody really has to die from a heart- or circulatory system-related death, it is even more of a tragedy. The disability, suffering, and years of life lost are almost totally the result of dietary ignorance. It is not impossible or even difficult to protect yourself; you simply must eat properly. Nothing else can protect you.

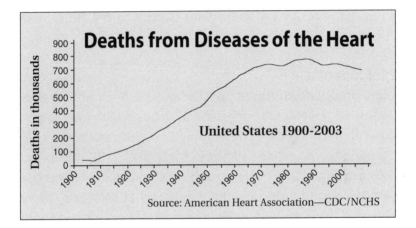

Are Americans living longer?

Most people accept the notion that we are living longer now than ever before in human history. This is not entirely true. The *average* age has gone up, but people who reach adulthood are not living longer than at other times in human history. Infant and childhood mortality has fallen dramatically.

Unlike in previous times, it is very rare today that a woman dies during or soon after childbirth. Modern plumbing and refrigeration methods have greatly lowered the rates of infectious diseases. However, adults do not have a longer healthy-life-expectancy than centuries ago because increases in the incidence of cancer, stroke, and heart disease have negated these advances in public health. The typical adult living today has almost no chance of reaching their genetic potential.

Diet and disease

Diets of all description flood the market, but fewer than 3 people out of 100 are successful at losing weight and keeping it off permanently. The number of overweight and obese individuals is at an all-time high and still climbing. Although many people accept the notion that disease is the result of genetics or luck, the reality is that nutrition, exercise, and environment overwhelmingly overshadow genetic considerations. For example, those living in rural China have less than a 2% heart disease risk, but when these same individuals move to America, their children develop the same rates of heart disease as other Americans.

Obviously, the diseases that afflict today's Americans are not the result of luck or genetics. They are a recent phenomenon in human history and directly parallel unhealthful

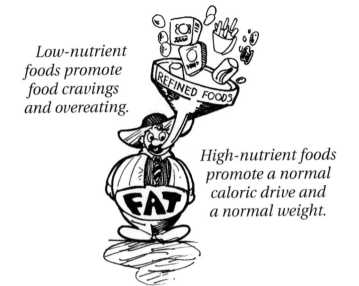

Low-nutrient foods promote food cravings and overeating.

High-nutrient foods promote a normal caloric drive and a normal weight.

changes in dietary patterns. The ten-fold increase in heart attacks in the last 100 years is because we are eating more low-nutrient food—lots more. You cannot escape from the biological law of cause and effect. Health results from healthful living and eating. Disease and premature death result primarily from unhealthful food choices.

Home cooking better
A major factor in the increase of diet-related health problems is the fact that Americans no longer make and eat most of their meals at home. The once common scene of a

family gathered around the kitchen eating a healthful home-cooked meal has become so rare that many of today's children have never experienced it. About half of all food dollars are spent eating outside the home, with the largest percent of this being spent in fast food restaurants. Traditional homemade foods are not only more healthful, they are lower in calories. Research shows that we consume *double* the calories when we eat out.

Macronutrients

Macronutrients are nutrients that contain calories. There are only three macronutrients—fat, carbohydrate, and protein. Macronutrients give us the calories we need for energy and growth. All natural foods contain a mixture of fat, carbohydrate, and protein, although some (primarily animal products) contain only two of the three. For example, a banana is mostly carbohydrate (93%), but it does contain some fat (3%) and protein (4%). Spinach, like all dark leafy green vegetables, contains approximately equal amounts of carbohydrate (40%) and protein (43%), along with a lesser amount of fat (7%). Sirloin steak is all fat (44%) and protein (56%) and contains no carbohydrate. I've listed a few more examples on the next page.

With Americans gaining weight at such a fast pace, there seems to be an endless stream of diet books that focus on

Macronutrient Percentages in 10 Sample Foods

Food	Carbohydrate	Fat	Protein
Frozen spinach	43.5	16.9	39.6
Artichokes	74.4	2.4	23.2
Sesame seeds	15.3	73.1	11.6
Red kidney beans	69.9	3.5	26.6
Whole wheat bread	71.4	16.9	11.7
Banana	92.6	3.0	4.4
Hot dog	2.3	82.4	15.3
Low-fat yogurt	64.1	13.1	22.9
Swiss cheese	5.7	65.9	28.4
Sirloin steak	0	44.0	56.0

manipulating the amounts and the percentages of the macronutrients—carbohydrate, fat, and protein—that we eat. But fiddling around with macronutrient percentages is not the way to lose weight or improve health. In fact, the only way to slow the tidal wave of increased chronic disease and obesity is for people to eat less of all three macronutrients.

It is a simple equation. Macronutrients are where all of the calories come from. If you overconsume macronutrients (regardless of the percentages of each), you will get too many calories. If you consume too many calories, you will experience excess weight gain, various chronic diseases, and premature death.

To lose weight and improve health, forget about macro-nutrient percentages, and focus on providing yourself with the highest *quality* diet. Nutritional excellence is achieved by eating foods that have the highest levels of *micro*nutrients.

Micronutrients

Micronutrients are essential nutritional substances that do not contain calories. The three main micronutrients are vitamins, minerals, and phytochemicals. (Some researchers consider fiber and water to be micronutrients, too.) Micro-nutrients are extremely important for your health.

Micronutrients are needed for your body to manufac-ture the materials it needs for normal function, to rid itself of waste, and to repair damage. Without micronutrients, you quickly would get sick and die soon afterwards. Americans eat too few micronutrients, and we would live longer if we ate more.

There are 13 vitamins and 25 minerals known to be important for human health, and the importance of the adequate intake of them for overall health cannot be over-stated. Their impact on overall health is broad and vast; the effects of deficiencies are devastating. The human body requires large amounts of some of them, and trace amounts of others. Natural foods have been shown to contain the right types of them in the right proportions for human survival and good health.

Unnatural foods

Knowing that the right micronutrients in the right proportions are easily available to us in whole, natural foods is wonderful. But we no longer get our foods in natural form from the wild. Most of the food we eat is concocted in factories. These processed foods do not contain the level and diversity of the vitamins and minerals we get in natural foods. For example, the fruits and vegetables that primates eat in the wild are loaded with micronutrients, giving these primates a diet far richer in many essential vitamins and minerals than the diets consumed by any humans in the modern world.

A study of monkey diets carried out at the University of California, Berkeley, by anthropologist Katharine Milton found, for instance, that the average 15-pound wild monkey takes in 600 milligrams per day of vitamin C, 10 times more than the 60-milligram recommended daily allowance (RDA) for the average 150-pound human. Differences on that order also were found for intakes of other micronutrients, such as fiber, magnesium, potassium, and beta-carotene. The monkey's diet is amazingly rich in nutrients. The foods that primates in the wild eat include green leaves of many kinds and fruits such as figs, plums, berries, and grapes. The study also reported that the dark green vegetables the monkeys eat contain the complete array of essential amino acids, similar to meat.

The RDAs set by the government were determined by investigating the foods modern humans eat, and they should not be considered representative of the amount of nutrients that would be found in an *ideal* diet. Unfortunately, most people don't even take in the very low levels recommended in the RDAs. The researchers in the monkey study concluded that "throughout history, humans have suffered from all sorts of diet-related diseases. If we paid more attention to what our wild, primate relatives are eating today, perhaps we could learn new things about our own dietary needs that would help reduce health problems throughout the world."

The modern diet, especially the one most Americans eat, is too low in minerals and not even close to what we should be consuming for optimal health. Despite consuming almost twice as many calories (macronutrients) as we need, fewer than 18% of adults and 2% of children consume the minimum daily requirement of micronutrients recommended.

Phytochemicals

As serious as deficiencies in vitamins and minerals have become, there is an even more serious one—deficiencies of phytochemicals.

There are over 1,000 important phytochemicals. Phytochemicals are the most recently found class of micronutrients, and they are necessary for your cells to remove waste and to maintain normal immune function. Fortunately, phytochemicals are present in foods that also are naturally high in vitamins and minerals (i.e., natural plant foods).

For optimal health, you need lots of phytochemicals in your diet. Consuming abundant amounts of micronutrients will help protect you against disease, and if you already are sick, it can help you recover. Vegetables, beans, and fruit are naturally high in micronutrients, but Americans don't eat much of them. We eat plenty of meat, cheese, chicken, pasta, white bread, oils, soda, and cookies, which are very low in micronutrients and contain no phytochemicals.

Poor nutrition and disease

Poor nutrition is the primary cause of common diseases. Since micronutrients are critical for the prevention of diseases such as heart disease, cancer, and dementia, it should be clear why these and other diseases have become so prevalent. For example, deaths due to diabetes have increased 45% since 1987. Diabetes is fueled by excess body fat and low nutrient levels in the body's tissues. The micronutrient deficiencies also leave the body prone to infections, allergies, headaches, fatigue, body aches, bowel problems, kidney diseases, arthritis, and emotional disorders.

About seventy-five years ago, scientists discovered vitamins and minerals and noted that diseases occurred when vitamin deficiencies occurred. It also was noted that low vitamin intake could lead to cancer. These discoveries led to the creation of the vitamin industry, which today supplies both synthetic vitamins and natural vitamins isolated from their original sources to food manufacturers and many other outlets. Unfortunately, trying to assure vitamin adequacy by adding synthetic supplements and isolated vitamins to a diet virtually devoid of the natural sources of these micronutrients did not turn out well. The cancer rate in America rose every year for seventy-five years straight (1930-2005).

About twenty years ago, researchers found the missing link. They discovered that colorful plant foods in their natural state were also rich in thousands of compounds with important health properties for humans—phytochemicals. Only by eating an assortment of natural foods that are micronutrient-rich can you get enough of these compounds to protect yourself from the common diseases that afflict Americans.

This new revelation in the science of health taught us that we need to eat a diet with lots of high-nutrient foods and that supplements cannot take the place of these foods. With this newfound knowledge, we have seen the power of nutritional excellence to prevent and even reverse disease. We have witnessed the power of micronutrients.

As you can see, we cannot expect the health of our nation to improve through medical interventions when the underlying cause of the problems—diets dangerously low in micronutrients that are essential to maximize human cellular function—is left unchanged.

Dietary-Induced Premature Aging

Effects of the typical American diet:
- *Excessive weight gain*
- *Diabetes and high blood pressure*
- *Hardening of arteries*
- *Increased LDL cholesterol*
- *Autoimmune diseases*
- *Cancer*

Low-nutrient foods

Just as eating large amounts of micronutrient-rich natural plant foods is of great benefit to your health, eating large amounts of micronutrient-deficient animal foods and processed foods leaves you very susceptible to disease. That is why the standard American diet (SAD) results in the diseases Americans get.

Neither animal products nor processed foods contain antioxidants, bioflavonoids, carotenoids, folate, vitamin C, or those thousands of phytochemicals that are essential for cellular normalcy. Many of the animal products consumed, such as cheese and red meat, are exceptionally high in saturated fat. High saturated fat intake increases the risk of certain cancers and promotes high cholesterol, leading to heart disease. To add insult to injury, many of the processed foods we eat are high in trans fat, a man-made fat that is linked to cancer and heart disease.

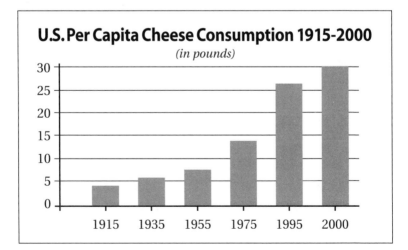

U.S. Per Capita Cheese Consumption 1915-2000
(in pounds)

Saturated Fat Content of Various Foods

Food	Fat content in grams
Cheddar cheese (4 oz.)	24
American processed cheese (4 oz.)	24
Ricotta cheese (1 cup)	20
Swiss cheese (4 oz.)	20
Chocolate candy, semisweet (4 oz.)	20
Cheeseburger, large double patty	18
T-bone steak (6 oz.)	18
Pork, shoulder (6 oz.)	14.5
Butter (2 Tbsp.)	14
Mozzarella, part skim (4 oz.)	12
Ricotta cheese, part skim (1 cup)	12
Beef, ground, lean (6 oz.)	11
Ice cream, vanilla (1 cup)	10
Chicken fillet sandwich	9
Chicken thigh, no skin (6 oz.)	5
Milk, whole, 3.3% fat (1 cup)	5
Plain yogurt	5
Two eggs	4
Chicken breast (6 oz.)	3
Salmon (6 oz.)	3
Milk, 2% fat (1 cup)	3
Tuna (6 oz.)	2.6
Turkey, white, no skin, (6 oz.)	2
Flounder or sole (6 oz.)	0.6
Fruits	negligible
Vegetables	negligible
Beans/legumes	negligible

A needless tragedy

Clearly, Americans are eating too much saturated fat and trans fat. Even worse, these fats become more dangerous when accompanied by lots of processed foods. Processed foods are made mostly of sugar, white flour, and oil, which contain almost no micronutrients. Micronutrient deficiencies caused by excess intake of saturated fat, animal protein, and salt and an inadequate intake of unrefined, high-nutrient plant foods lead to a potent disease-promoting synergy that is the primary cause of most life-shortening diseases in America.[1] You could not have designed a better environment for creating cancer and heart attacks if you scientifically planned it. Because of the poor food choices being made by most Americans, our country is suffering from extremely high instances of chronic illnesses, and our healthcare costs are spiraling out of control.

The standard low-nutrient diet consumed by most Americans results in fatty deposits in the walls of the blood vessels that eventually lead to blood vessel narrowing and blood clots that cause strokes and heart attacks. The disease-building process is not the by-product of aging; rather it is the by-product of a diet that is poorly designed for human primates. The micronutrient deficiencies gradually lead to more and more damage as time goes on. This disease process of decreased blood flow and the resulting

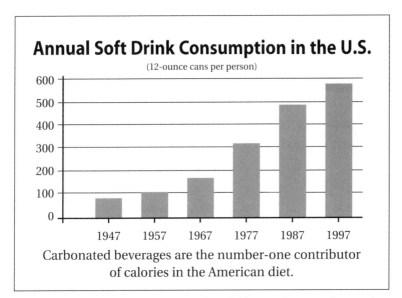

Annual Soft Drink Consumption in the U.S.
(12-ounce cans per person)

Carbonated beverages are the number-one contributor
of calories in the American diet.

diminished nutrient delivery should be understood as a single disease process, one that can be remedied by removing
the original cause—poor diet. Unfortunately, this singular
cause and effect is obscured by the way diseases are
named—based on which organ shows the most serious (or
most obvious) symptoms. Thus, for example, heart attacks
and angina (diseased blood vessels in the heart), high blood
pressure and strokes (diseased blood vessels leading to and
in the brain), dementia (diseased blood vessels in the
brain), impotence (diseased blood vessels leading to and in
the penis), and claudication (diseased blood vessels in the

legs) are treated as individual diseases, when in fact they are merely different manifestations of the same disease.

Unprecedented opportunity

Advances in nutritional and health sciences have given us an unprecedented opportunity to be healthier, to live longer than ever before, to disease-proof our bodies, and to add many quality years to our lives. Scientific studies have demonstrated that the damage to diseased blood vessels can be gradually reversed, and the damaged blood vessels can become unclogged.[2] The "secret" is to eat large quantities of high-nutrient foods.

Nutritional excellence is the secret to optimal health, disease prevention, and maintaining a healthy, slim waistline. In fact, it is the *only* way to lose weight healthfully and permanently. Everything else, such as magic drinks, fat-binding pills, energy boosters, herbal picker-uppers, and those cancer-causing high-protein diets, is doomed to failure. Instead of looking for magic, commit yourself to a new, healthy you. Most diseases are effectively treated through nutritional means and, in many cases, are completely reversed through aggressive nutritional intervention.

Chapter Two

Dramatic Results Without Drugs

If you desire to throw away your medications and recover from chronic illnesses such as heart disease, high blood pressure, and diabetes (all examples of common illnesses that are more effectively treated with nutritional intervention than drugs or surgery) and get slim at the same time, then nutritional excellence is the most effective approach. I have studied the results of nutritional intervention on thousands of my own patients, and the results have been dramatic. For example, I have helped thousands of patients successfully lower their cholesterol levels *without drugs.*

Just as an example, one day recently I saw four patients who dropped their LDL cholesterol below 100 mg/dl. Remember, this was just *one day* in my practice! Not only did each of these patients previously have dangerously high cholesterols, but each also had reported numerous additional health problems. Peggy suffered from chronic anemia. Eugene was tired all the time. Keith had chronic heartburn and allergies. Maria had become severely ill from a statin drug prescribed to her by her prior physician. These four patients needed help, and they realized that prescription drugs were risky and not the answer. They all returned to my office between 6 and 8 weeks after their first visit, and this is what we found.

	Before	*After*
Peggy:		
Total cholesterol	249	150
Triglycerides	169	105
LDL	157	80
HDL	58	49
Eugene:		
Total cholesterol	247	156
Triglycerides	72	42
LDL	191	104
HDL	51	44
Keith:		
Total cholesterol	237	158
Triglycerides	165	79
LDL	152	99
HDL	52	43.5

	Before	*After*
Maria:		
Total cholesterol	283	168
Triglycerides	90	79
LDL	183	98
HDL	91	52

Not only did they wipe out their cardiovascular high-risk status, but many of their other problems also began to clear. Peggy's anemia went away. Eugene was no longer fatigued. Keith never had heartburn again. He stopped his antacids and acid-blocking medication, and his allergies started to improve. Maria recovered from her severe illness from the statin drug. They all became enthusiastic about life again.

When you adopt a program of nutritional excellence to reverse or prevent heart disease, you experience a tremendously beneficial side effect—you will prevent and reverse almost all other diseases simultaneously. For example, you will likely find your digestion improves, and your heartburn, hemorrhoids, constipation, and headaches will disappear, too. You'll gain more energy, age more slowly, and your risk of other serious diseases—especially dementia, strokes, diabetes, and cancer—will decrease.

There have been cases where a patient has had to overcome some discomforting dietary hurdles after switching from a dairy-meat-processed food diet to one that is vegetable-fruit based and rich in nutrients and phytochemicals. But those symptoms are temporary. All of the patients who make the switch enjoy eating this new way. They learn to enjoy the new tastes and aromas and their newfound energy, and it motivates them to take steps to enjoy healthier and more fulfilling lives.

Great results like those achieved by Peggy, Eugene, Keith, and Maria are not limited only to patients who live near enough to come see me in my office. Hardly a day goes by when I do not receive an e-mail or letter from someone who tells me about the success he or she has achieved. This letter from Joe in Connecticut is typical.

Dear Dr. Fuhrman,

My name is Joe Lavaler, and I am one happy 68-year-old. I have generally enjoyed relatively good health over the years. However, I have struggled with high blood pressure (160/105) and high cholesterol (275) for many years. My cardiologist visit last October resulted in his increasing my Lipitor from 10mg/day to 20mg/day. Also, he placed me on Accupril. I told him that I had recently bought your tape and book, *Eat to Live,* and that I was going to make a major diet change and follow your recommendations instead. I have been following your program since November 2002 with spectacular results, and I have been able to stop all medications. I saw my cardiologist yesterday, and here are the results of my blood work:

Total cholesterol	148
Triglycerides	85
LDL	69
HDL	62

While my weight had been constant since high school at 235 pounds (I am 6'6" tall), I currently weigh 211 lbs. and feel better than I have in a long time. My wife and I cook most days in a Crock-Pot. We make a lot of soups with collard greens, mustard greens, spinach, beans, etc. I tell everyone who will listen that there is no "free lunch" and that you have to stay focused and committed.

My cardiologist, Dr. Kunkes, of Fairfield, Connecticut, said I made a remarkable turnaround and should be proud of myself. I brought a copy of your book with me. He said that he had heard of your program. He copied your web address and said he was planning on reading your book. I want to thank you for my greatly improved health. I would be willing to talk to any of your patients to help give them the support and encouragement they need to stay with the program. It worked where all other diets failed.

Sincerely yours,
Joseph Lavaler

Removing causes, not symptoms

Uncovering the causes of a health problem, and eliminating them when possible, always results in a more favorable outcome than simply covering up symptoms with medications. When you eat foods that are naturally rich in micronutrients, it helps control overeating, and the lower caloric intake enables your body to more effectively undertake its self-healing tasks. Countless studies have shown that the combination of high-nutrient intake and lower caloric intake promotes disease-resistance and longevity. In addition to reducing the occurrence of cancer and heart disease, high-micronutrient diets reduce the occurrence of cataracts, dementia, kidney stones, gout, osteoarthritis, back pain, diabetes, and depression. Adopting a better diet could dramatically increase your health, productivity, and life span.

Increasing your consumption of high-nutrient fruits and vegetables is the key to disease resistance, disease reversal, and a long, healthy life. The potential reduction in disease rates shows no threshold effect in the scientific studies. That means that as high-nutrient vegetables and high-nutrient fruits increase as a major portion of caloric intake, disease rates fall in a dose-dependent manner—the more the diet is comprised of these foods, the better your health will be.[3]

The recommendations presented in this book will help

you if you are looking to stay well and maintain your youthful vigor, free of the chronic diseases that plague so many Americans. But to live longer and more healthfully, you must *Eat To Live.*

The science and logic behind *Eat to Live* and my two-book set, *Eat For Health*, is easy to understand. It is not based on narrow or obscure scientific principles; rather it is based on the preponderance of evidence from thousands of scientific studies. The result is an opportunity, unprecedented in human history, to achieve superior health with a comprehensive program based on the nutrient density of foods.

Dr. Fuhrman's Health Equation
$$H = N/C$$
Health = Nutrient intake divided by Calorie intake

Do you agree that your body builds and repairs itself using the food you eat? Do you agree that high-quality, high-nutrient food makes a high-quality body that is more resistant to the diseases that are ravaging our nation? I hope you do because all of the leading nutritional scientists the world over have accepted these basic concepts. In a nutshell, you are what you eat.

There are distinct advantages to choosing healthful,

nutrient-rich foods over unhealthful, nutrient-poor ones. If you want those advantages, I urge you to become familiar with my simple Health Equation: H = N/C. This equation is a powerful tool that can predict whether your eating habits are putting you at risk of a serious disease such as heart attack or stroke and shortening your life span. Using it helps you make food choices that can help you to maintain youthful vigor and mental capacity as you age.

The Health Equation: H = N/C illustrates the concept that to be in excellent health, your diet must be high in nutrients (micronutrients), and you must not overeat on calories. Another way of saying that is your health is dependent on the nutrient-to-calorie ratio of your diet. If you agree (as leading researchers do) that the nutrient density in your body's tissues is proportional to the nutrient density of your diet, then you must accept the fact that to be healthy and disease-resistant you need to eat more high-nutrient foods and fewer low-nutrient foods.

Permanently maintaining healthy weight

Temporary weight-loss techniques (what we all call "dieting") serve no purpose. There is no health benefit to losing weight and then putting it back on again soon afterwards. Health benefits only occur when the weight loss is maintained *forever*. That means that the only dietary change that

Weight and Diabetes

O besity is closely associated with more than seventeen major chronic conditions, including heart disease, cancer, and diabetes. Researchers base their definition of obesity on body mass index (BMI), the ratio between weight and height.

Diabetes is a good example of how the incidence of serious disease goes up as your weight increases.

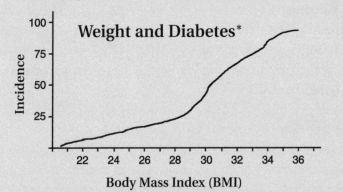

As you can see on the chart, as BMI index rises above 25, the incidence of diabetes increases rapidly. At a BMI of 25, diabetes risk is 15%. At a BMI of 30, risk increases to 50%. By the time BMI reaches 35, risk is a staggering 90%.

Similar increases occur with other chronic diseases.

* Diabetes Care 2007;30(6):1562-66.

can work is one that you stick with permanently. If the change you make to your diet is permanent, you are not on a diet; you merely have changed your eating habits.

Eating more high-nutrient food is the only way to lose weight permanently, and eating more nutrients leads to permanent improvements in your health. Knowing these important facts and *putting them into practice* is your key to health and longevity. Fortunately, eating more high-nutrient foods helps control food cravings and overeating behaviors, making it easier to reach your ideal weight. This knowledge can guide you for the rest of your life. It is not a fad, and it will never go out of style. High-nutrient eating is the way of the future, but you can enjoy it now. It can be your fountain of youth.

How nutrients control your appetite

Hunger is a complicated thing. It is controlled by a system of messengers—hormones, nerves, and neurotransmitters. When your body's micronutrient needs are not met, you can be driven to eat more calories than you need for optimal health.

Because of poor diet and health habits, many people experience uncomfortable symptoms a few hours after eating. This leads them to eat too often—and too much—as a way of preventing the discomfort. The symptoms are similar to those drug addicts feel when they are too long without their "fix." Like drug addicts, people with food addictions feel poorly after digestion because their bodies are experiencing withdrawal symptoms. Since eating again (akin to taking another "fix") makes the discomfort go away, these detoxification symptoms are mistaken for hunger. I call these symptoms "toxic hunger." Toxic hunger goes away when you establish the habit of eating a high-nutrient diet.

Symptoms of toxic hunger
- *Shakes*
- *Headaches*
- *Lightheadedness*
- *Stomach fluttering*
- *Abdominal cramping*
- *Mental confusion*

Be forewarned. Eating healthfully may make the symptoms of toxic hunger feel worse temporarily. When you stop drinking coffee or discontinue other harmful habits, you may experience withdrawal or detox symptoms for a week or so. However, in a short time these long-standing symptoms will disappear, and you will not be driven to overeat anymore. You quickly will become comfortable eating less, and you will no longer desire the extra calories you used to crave to palliate unpleasant symptoms.

After a period of time eating a diet much higher in micronutrients, you eventually will experience what I call true hunger, which is felt mostly in the throat. It can direct you to the appropriate amount of calories—not too many and not too few. One of the huge benefits of high-nutrient eating is that you lose the food cravings, hypoglycemic symptoms, and other sensations that drive people to overeat. You will become more in touch with your body's natural instinctive signals, and you will know when, what, and how much to eat. You will know when food is really needed. These natural, true hunger signals will help direct you to your ideal body weight. You will be able to step off the dieting merry-go-round.

H = N/C is not only the secret formula for health, it also is the best formula for weight loss. As you eat higher on the

Start Eating a Higher-Nutrient Diet!

The best way to begin improving your diet is to focus more on eating *micronutrients* and less on eating *macronutrients*.

See page 83 to learn about Dr. Fuhrman's Top 30 Super Foods with the highest nutrient density.

Eat more micronutrients: vitamins, minerals, phytochemicals, fiber.

Eat fewer macronutrients: protein, carbohydrates, fat.

nutrient chart and take in high levels of phytochemicals, you will find yourself effortlessly losing weight without dieting. Eating for nutritional excellence is the only sensible way to diet. There is only one best way to eat for better health and a thinner you, and that is to eat a diet rich in micronutrients.

Silent, invisible damage

We continually are being told that heart disease, high cholesterol, high blood pressure, and even dementia are the inevitable consequences of aging. So it is not surprising that most people assume that we have to expect these things as they are. We also are told that they are primarily the result of genetics and, therefore, are beyond our control. The statistics seemingly bear this out. Over 90% percent of elderly Americans require medications for high blood pressure or other heart conditions. But these diseases are not the consequence of aging; they are the consequence of consuming a low-nutrient diet over time.

We don't see the harm as we hurt our bodies in tiny increments, day after day, by eating a low-nutrient diet. Children, teenagers, and young adults "seem" to get away with years of poor nutrition. But after enough time goes by, the damage is easily seen. Then, we blame it on aging.

Let me illustrate my point with one of my patients, John Pawlokoski. When John first came to me as a patient in 1994, he was age 69. He reported that he first experienced pain in his chest and arms while exerting himself working in his backyard. He soon began to get uncomfortable with minimal activity, and he was given medications, including calcium channel blockers and nitroglycerin, to relieve his symptoms. He saw a cardiologist who performed a stress thallium and a cardiac catherization that demonstrated four areas of severe narrowing. Angioplasty was recommended.

John in 1994 at age 69

Weight	180
Blood pressure	160/90
Cholesterol	240
LDL cholesterol	156
Glucose	98
Medications	2 blood pressure medications, 1 cholesterol-lowering drug, nitroglycerin

Following his evaluation with me, John decided to follow my nutritional advice 100%. Within two months he had lost 14 pounds, and he had no further angina (chest pain) symptoms. He did not need to use nitroglycerin any longer and was able to be active and exercise without symptoms.

After the first month, his total cholesterol dropped to 168. He saw his cardiologist again. The cardiologist agreed that since John was using an effective dietary approach that was working so well, there was no need to go forward with the angioplasty. John never had a heart or health problem again. His blood pressure became lower and lower with each passing month on the high-nutrient diet, and his cholesterol dropped further and further. He was able to discontinue all drugs. He ate himself to wellness.

John in 2006 at age 81

Weight	150
Blood pressure	95/70
Cholesterol	140
LDL cholesterol	70
Glucose	68
Medications	none

I told you about John to illustrate what I observe with all of my patients. They get healthier the longer they stay on the healthful diet, and their diseases slowly melt away with time. As John got older, he got healthier. High blood pressure, high cholesterol, and the resultant diseases they cause were not from aging. John's disease parameters got lower and lower with time, until he reached his ideal weight and his ideal blood pressure and cholesterol. His own body provided the "cure" when it was supplied with the right raw materials to work with. You can get well, too, no matter what your age!

Your body is a miraculous self-healing machine when your nutritional needs are met. You can protect yourself not just from heart disease, but also from many other diseases, such as diabetes, cancer, strokes, senility, and dementia. You can get healthier and healthier every day. Like John, you can control your health destiny.

The real fountain of youth

Most Americans have given up hope of ever achieving their optimal weight and health. They have failed with diets in the past. They think they can't lose weight, and they don't think they can change. So they just throw in the towel. By now, you should be beginning to understand why those diets failed and why they became too difficult to stick with. At this point, you have a choice to make. Do you want to develop the common diseases that other Americans do and flirt with a premature death? Or do you want to enjoy good health as you age gracefully?

I know that there will be people reading this who will be thinking, *I know eating vegetables and fruits is healthy, but I don't want to eat like that. I enjoy unhealthful food too much, and I would rather die young than not enjoy my food.* If you are one of them, here are a few more things you may not have considered. The first is that your taste adjusts, and you begin to relish the new foods once you get used to eating them. The second is that you can quickly learn how to make high-nutrient food taste so great that you think you are eating in a 5-star gourmet restaurant. This is not primarily a recipe book (although there are some great ones starting on page 63), but have no fear—great tasting healthful recipes abound. Visit www.EatRightAmerica.com for information on how to purchase my comprehensive two-book set, *Eat For Health,* one volume of which is devoted *entirely* to recipes.

Now you can enjoy great tasting food and add 20 or more healthful years to your life. I guarantee you that if you learn more and follow this program faithfully, you soon will enjoy eating more—not less—than you do now.

Now that you know you can control your health destiny through high-nutrient eating, let's take a look at high-nutrient eating in action. Learn the foods that are richest in micronutrients, and then I will show you how to plan a menu with recipes that will disease-proof your body.

Chapter Three

Measuring Nutrient Density

Nutrient density is a critical concept in devising and recommending dietary and nutritional advice to patients and to the public. Micronutrient density and diversity are essential for a normal immune system and for the detoxification and cellular repair mechanisms that protect you from cancer and other diseases.

Our modern American, low-nutrient diet leads to an overweight population suffering from the common diseases of nutritional ignorance and a national medical bill that is spiraling out of control. High-nutrient eating has the opposite effect. When you ingest a broader assortment and amount of these phytochemicals, your body functions better and resists the effects of "aging." Nutritional excellence also helps minimize any genetic weaknesses you may have. Phytochemicals are necessary to enable your body's defenses against cancer and cardiovascular disease, the leading causes of death in the modern world.

To be able to eat more of the foods that are high in nutrients and fewer of the foods that are low in nutrients, you must learn which foods are which. Once you know the nutrient scores of foods, you will be able to make better choices as you shop and eat. As you eat more high-nutrient foods and minimize your consumption of low-nutrient foods, you will see dramatic health benefits.

The nutrient density rankings of foods in this book are derived from Dr. Fuhrman's Aggregate Nutrient Density Index* (ANDI), which is described on page 85. The rankings in this book can supplement the high-nutrient hierarchy explained in my book, *Eat to Live,* and in my comprehensive two-book set, *Eat For Health.* (For more information, visit: www.EatRightAmerica.com). I encourage you to use these additional resources to further understand the science, logic, and application of my approach, and also to get a deeper understanding of the benefits of eating a diet that is higher in nutrient density. In addition, they will give you many valuable tips and strategies designed to make eating right pleasurable and delicious.

Because phytochemicals are largely unnamed and unmeasured, these rankings underestimate the healthful properties of colorful natural plant foods compared to processed foods and animal products. Fortunately, the foods

* Patent Pending

that contain the highest amounts of known nutrients also are the same foods that contain the most unknown nutrients. So even though these rankings may result in lower ratings for the highest-nutrient foods, they are still reasonable measurements of nutrient content.

Smart choices

In chapter 8, there are nutrient scores for a wide range of commonly eaten foods, including some high in saturated fat, trans fat, cholesterol, and added salt. These are not recommended foods and are included simply to help people make choices as they make the transition to nutritional excellence.

Since the foods with the higher nutrient scores are low in calories and do not contain saturated fat, trans fat, cholesterol, or added salt, you need not give these unhealthful food factors much thought once you start choosing foods that have the highest nutrient density. For example, all natural foods contain less than half a mg of sodium per calorie.

It is only when you include prepared foods, processed foods, and restaurant foods in your diet that excess sodium becomes an issue (because of the risk of high blood pressure and strokes). When eating foods from lower-nutrient categories, the sodium levels need to be considered.

Try to avoid foods with more salt than calories. Foods that contain more sodium (in milligrams) than the number of calories cannot be considered healthful. As the sodium number gets higher and higher, the food becomes more dangerous to include in your diet. Ideally, your total daily intake of sodium should be under 1000 mg.

Sample scores

Below is a sample list of nutrient scores for some familiar foods. There are additional comparisons that appear later in this book, as well as a comprehensive list of nutrient scores for foods commonly eaten in America. The higher the number, the better the food.

Sample Nutrient/Calorie Density Scores

Dr. Fuhrman's Aggregate Nutrient Density Index* (ANDI)

The higher the number, the better the food.

Kale	1000	Broccoli	342
Collards	1000	Cauliflower	295
Watercress	1000	Green pepper	258
Bok choy	824	Tomato sauce	247
Spinach (uncooked)	697	Artichoke	244
Brussels sprouts	672	Carrots	240
Swiss chard	670	Asparagus	234
Arugula	559	Strawberries	212
Radish	554	Pomegranate juice	193
Cabbage (cooked)	481	Tomato	164
Bean sprouts	444	Plums	157
Red pepper	420	Raspberries	145
Romaine lettuce	389	Blueberries	130

Brazil nuts	117	Walnuts	29
Iceberg lettuce	110	Pistachio nuts	29
Orange	109	Chicken breast	27
Grapefruit	102	Egg	27
Cantaloupe	100	Low-fat plain yogurt	26
Tofu	86	Shredded wheat	26
Sweet potato	84	Whole wheat bread	25
Apple	76	Corn	25
Peach	74	Almonds	24
Green peas	70	Feta cheese	21
Cherries	68	Milk chocolate	21
Kidney beans	56	Whole milk	20
Oatmeal	53	Ground beef	20
Mango	51	Dates	19
Cucumber	50	Whole wheat pasta	19
Soybeans	48	White bread	18
Prunes	47	Peanut butter	18
Sunflower seeds	46	White pasta	18
Shrimp	45	Raisins	17
Flaxseed	44	Cashews	16
Sesame seeds	41	Apple juice	16
Brown rice	41	Swiss cheese	15
Salmon	39	Low-fat fruit yogurt	14
Avocado	37	White rice	12
Pork loin	37	Potato chips	11
Pumpkin seeds	36	Saltines	11
Skim milk	36	Vanilla ice cream	7
Pecans	34	Sugar cookies	5
Potato	32	Corn oil	3
Grapes	31	Olive oil	2
Cod	31	Honey	1
Banana	30	Cola	.5

Multifaceted needs

Keep in mind that nutrient density scoring is not the only factor that determines good health, and you should eat some of your diet from lower-nutrient categories. For example, if you only ate foods with the very highest nutrient density score, your diet could be too low in calories or too low in fat.

The percentage of fat intake can vary from 15-40% on a healthful diet, depending on the percentage of higher-fat fare such as avocados and raw nuts and seeds eaten as a percentage of total calories. Eating more of these higher-calorie, higher-fat foods is necessary for an active, thin person, athlete, or growing child. If an avid (or professional) athlete ate only the very highest-nutrient foods, she would become too full from all of the food volume and fiber, and so satiated from the *micro*nutrient fulfillment, that it could keep her from meeting her caloric (*macro*nutrient) needs. She could become too thin. This, of course, gives you a hint at the secret to permanent weight control. "Dieting" is not needed to maintain a healthful weight. You only need to eat more high-nutrient food and less low-nutrient food. The most healthful way to lose weight is to increase the overall nutrient density of your diet. The more high-nutrient foods you eat, the thinner you get.

As you will see, some categories of foods are lower in

nutrient density than others. When selecting foods from those categories, pick from the higher-nutrient foods in each category.

Misconceptions about protein

The most common question people are asked when they switch to a nutrient-rich diet is, "Where do you get your protein?" In a diet that is chock-full of vegetables and fruits, and short on animal products, it might seem like a reasonable question. But it isn't.

It is an old myth that a diet needs to contain lots of animal products to provide enough protein and be nutritionally sound. Adding to the confusion are diet books and magazine articles that promulgate another myth—that eating more protein is weight-loss favorable and eating carbohydrates is weight-loss unfavorable. Another common misconception is the notion that you need to maintain a fixed, exact ratio (percentage) of fat, carbohydrate, and protein. There also are plenty of self-appointed experts ready to tell you that the ideal diet should be based on your heritage, skin tone, eye color, blood type, or the spelling of your mother's maiden name. Some recommend high-protein, others low-protein; some recommend very low-fat diets; others recommend much higher levels of fat. But regulating the macro-nutrient content of a diet is not the critical factor you should be concerned with, and here's why.

If you are overweight, you have consumed more calories than you have utilized. Micromanaging the percent of fat, protein, or carbohydrate isn't going to change the amount of calories very much. You need to consume fewer calories. Therefore, almost all overweight individuals need to consume less of all the macronutrients—less protein, less fat, and less carbohydrate. These are the source of all calories. Don't worry about not consuming enough of any of these. Unless you are anorexic, it is very rare to find an American who is deficient in fat, protein, or carbohydrates.

There is protein in all foods, *especially vegetables,* not just in animal products. The fact is, protein deficiency is not a concern for anyone in the developed world. It is almost impossible to consume too little protein, no matter what you eat, unless your diet is significantly deficient in overall calories. If it is, you'll be deficient in other nutrients as well.

It is a big mistake to put emphasis on trying to get enough of something (protein) you are undoubtedly getting too much of in the first place. Hundreds of studies show that as protein consumption goes up, so does the incidence of chronic diseases. Is protein bad for us? No, incidence of chronic diseases goes up when you increase the consumption of carbohydrates and fat, too.[4] Most Americans simply don't need to increase eating any macronutrients. Increasing the consumption of protein (or fat or carbohydrates) is good if you need more calories because you are anorexic or are chronically malnourished, like a starving person in a troubled area of the world. But it is bad if you are already getting too much. If any of these nutrients exceed our basic requirements, the excess is harmful. Americans already get too much protein, and it is hurting us.[5]

The problem is that people in modern societies like the United States eat diets that are deficient in *micro*nutrients, not macronutrients. The focus of this book is to promote the consumption of high-micronutrient food. Simply put, the goal of a high-level diet is to get the most micronutrients, in both amount and diversity, from the fewest calories. H = N/C.

Key to superior health and your ideal weight

When you eat to maximize micronutrients in relation to calories, your body functions will normalize; chronic illnesses such as high blood pressure, diabetes, and high cholesterol melt away; and you maintain your youthful vigor into old age. Heart disease and cancer would fade away and become exceedingly rare if people adopted a lifestyle of nutritional excellence. But in the here and now, what is exciting to so many people is that when your diet is high enough in micronutrients, excess weight drops off at a relatively fast rate. It's like you had your stomach stapled. You simply don't crave to overeat anymore. In fact, it becomes too difficult to overeat when you eat your fill of high-micro-nutrient food.

The mistake of focusing on the "importance" of protein in the diet is one of the major reasons Americans have been led down the path to dietary suicide. For too long, we have equated protein with good nutrition and have thought that animal products—in spite of the fact that they are deficient or devoid of most micronutrients—are highly favorable foods simply because they are rich in complete proteins. This miscalculation has cost us dearly. By favoring a dairy- and meat-heavy diet, instead of one rich in fruits, vegetables, and beans, we have brought forth an epidemic of heart attacks and cancers.

Complete protein

When you hear something over and over from the time you were a young child, it is easy to accept it as true. So it should not come as a surprise that the myth that we need to consume animal products to get adequate protein is still alive and well in America. The myth that plant proteins are "incomplete" and need to be "complemented" for adequate protein is still alive, too.

Amino acids are the building blocks that make proteins.

All vegetables and grains contain all eight of the essential amino acids (as well as the twelve other non-essential ones). While some vegetables have higher or lower proportion of certain amino acids than others, when eaten in amounts to satisfy your caloric needs, a sufficient amount of all essential amino acids is provided. Today's nutritional science has deemphasized the importance of protein because we now know that it is easy to get enough, and that too much is not good.

Scientific studies on human protein requirements demonstrate that adults require 20-35 grams of protein per day.[6] Today, the average American consumes 100-120 grams of protein per day, mostly in the form of animal products. This high level of animal product consumption has been linked to not just heart disease and strokes, but to higher rates of cancer, as well.[7] We simply don't need all this protein. Even people who eat a total vegetarian (vegan) diet, which contains no animal products, have been found to consume 60-80 grams of protein per day, well above the minimum requirement.[8]

Plant protein and micronutrients

Eating more plant protein is the key to increasing our micronutrient intake. It is interesting to note that foods such as peas, green vegetables, and beans have lots of protein—even more protein per calorie than meat. But what is not generally considered is that foods that are rich in plant protein are generally the foods that are richest in nutrients and phytochemicals. By eating more of these high-nutrient, low-calorie foods, we get plenty of protein, and our bodies get flooded with protective micronutrients simultaneously. Animal protein does not contain antioxidants and phyto-chemicals; plant protein does. Plus, animal protein is married to saturated fat. Excesses of saturated fat are not favorable for good health.

Protein content of selected plant foods

Foods	Grams
Almonds (3 oz.)	10
Banana	1.2
Broccoli (two cups)	10
Brown rice (one cup)	5
Chickpeas (one cup)	15
Corn (one cup)	4.2
Lentils (one cup)	18
Peas, frozen (one cup)	9
Spinach, frozen (one cup)	7
Tofu (4 oz.)	11
Whole wheat bread (2 slices)	5

No complicated formulas or protein supplements are needed for you to get sufficient protein for growth, even if you are a serious athlete. Exercise drives an increased hunger, and as you consume more calories to meet the demands of exercise, you will naturally get the extra protein you need.

Weight loss and cholesterol

When you drop body fat, your cholesterol lowers some-what. But when you reduce animal protein intake and increase vegetable protein intake, your cholesterol lowers dramatically. In fact, when a high-fiber, high-nutrient, veg-etable-heavy diet was tested in a scientific investigation, it was found to lower cholesterol even more than most cho-lesterol-lowering drugs.[9] As you eat more vegetables and fewer animal products, the nutrient density of your diet will go up automatically. Vegetables not only contain adequate protein, they have no saturated fat or cholesterol, and they are higher in nutrients per calorie than any other food. You can achieve your ideal weight and slow the aging process with a high phytochemical intake. So eat more vegetables!

The cholesterol-lowering effects of vegetables and beans (high-protein foods) are without question. However, they contain an assortment of additional heart disease-fighting nutrients independent of their ability to lower cholesterol.[10] They fight cancer, too. Cancer incidence world-wide has an inverse relation with fruit and vegetable intake.[11] If you increase your intake 80%, the risk of getting cancer drops 80%.

Choose health

I urge you to start eating a diet that contains more high-nutrient plant foods today. Eat fewer animal products and fewer processed foods, and replace these calories with more fruits, vegetables, seeds, nuts, and beans. At minimum, I recommend that you cut back on animal-product consumption from three servings a day to one serving a day. Better yet, when you use animal products, add them to a dish in small amounts like condiments so that the total amount you consume each week will be even less. Eat vegetarian dinners frequently.

Make this dietary transition an exciting adventure where you learn new great-tasting recipes with high-nutrient plant foods. Design a food plan that uses large quantities of the most powerful anticancer, disease-fighting foods on the planet, make it taste great, and then test it to see what kinds of results you get. I can tell you now that the results will astound you!

Chapter Four

You Are What You Eat!

I f you need to lose weight, grasp the concept that being overweight has mostly to do with what you eat, not how much you eat. This is because micronutrient fulfillment (getting your fill of vitamins, minerals, phytochemicals, and fiber) blunts the drive to consume calories. Eating primarily high-nutrient foods is nothing like being on a "diet" (where you try to eat less). First of all, you will be eating hearty portions of (low-calorie) food. But most importantly, high-nutrient foods are so nutritionally satisfying that you simply will have less desire for the high-calorie, low-nutrient foods that put the weight on in the first place.

I hope it is clear that I am not advocating that you eat primarily high-nutrient foods for a period of time to lose weight and then go back to your old eating habits. I am advocating that you eat primarily high-nutrient foods from now on. The common practice of losing weight for a temporary period of time and then gaining it back is of no benefit to your health. Good health is dependent on maintaining a stable lighter weight for the rest of your life. That means you should *not* diet. What you should do is learn to eat a nutrient-rich diet, which will automatically reset your weight to a lower point permanently.

High-nutrient menus

Let's compare three days of menus. I've listed nutritionally excellent meals beside meals that are typical of the standard American diet. Each menu is followed by an analysis of its nutrient content and its total nutrient score. The differences are quite dramatic.

To show that even small changes can make a big difference, I've given examples of three progressively higher levels of nutritional excellence in the following menu comparisons. Nutritional excellence brings substantial benefits; the higher the nutrient density level, the more benefits you receive.

These three menus are merely a sample of the comprehensive nutritional makeover program described in my two-book set—*Eat For Health*. The complete *Eat For Health* program includes four phases of dietary excellence and 30 days of gourmet recipes.

To purchase the complete two-book set, *Eat For Health,* visit: www.EatRightAmerica.com or call: (877) ERA-4-USA.

Menu I Comparison

Standard American Diet vs. Eat For Health Diet

Standard American Diet

Breakfast
- Orange juice
- Cheerios
- Whole milk

Lunch
- Ham & cheese sandwich on roll w/ mayo
- Potato chips
- Coke

Dinner
- Crackers w/ cheese spread
- Spaghetti and meatballs
- Vanilla ice cream

Eat For Health Diet

Breakfast
- Fresh squeezed orange juice
- Oatmeal w/ blueberries, apples & nuts

Lunch
- Turkey sandwich on whole grain bread w/ mixed greens & tomato
- Strawberries
- Water

Dinner
- Tasty Hummus w/ Baked Garlic Pita Chips and raw veggies*
- Pasta w/ Roasted Vegetables*
- Creamy Banana Fig Ice Cream*

See Menu I Nutrient Analysis on the next page.

* See recipes in Chapter 5, beginning on p. 63.

Menu I Nutritional Analysis
Standard American Diet vs. Eat For Health Diet

	SAD	EFH
Calories	2011	1942
Protein	78	71
Carbohydrate	249	382
Fat	84	29
Cholesterol (mg)	337	20
Saturated fat	38	4
Fiber	15	54
Sodium (mg)	3660	1582
Vitamin C (mg)	183	603
B_1, thiamine (mg)	1.8	2.7
B_6, pyridoxine (mg)	1.3	2.8
Iron (mg)	23	23
Folate (ug)	409	802
Magnesium (mg)	148	491
Calcium	890	681
Zinc (mg)	8.7	8.9
Selenium (ug)	89	122
Alpha tocopherol (mg)	3.2	7.5
Beta-carotene (ug)	120	10,339
Alpha-carotene (ug)	15	2782
Lutein & zeaxanthin (ug)	300	1310
Lycopene (ug)	0	3532
Total Nutrient Score	*26*	*55*

Menu II Comparison
Standard American Diet vs. Eat For Health Diet

Standard American Diet

Breakfast
- Blueberry muffin
- Coffee/cream

Lunch
- Nachos w/ cheese
- Cookies

Dinner
- Iceburg lettuce salad w/Italian dressing
- Fried chicken
- French fries
- Corn
- Cake

Eat For Health Diet

Breakfast
- Blueberry Orange Smoothie*

Lunch
- Vegetable Bean Burrito*
- Apple

Dinner
- Mixed greens w/ Orange Cashew Dressing*
- Chicken Dijon*
- Baked Sweet Potato Fries*
- California Creamed Kale*
- Mango Coconut Sorbet*

See Menu II Nutrient Analysis on the next page.

* See recipes in Chapter 5, beginning on p. 63.

Menu II Nutritional Analysis
Standard American Diet vs. Eat For Health Diet

	SAD	EFH
Calories	2030	2086
Protein	81	103
Carbohydrate	217	271
Fat	96	79
Cholesterol (mg)	277	148
Saturated fat	32	13
Fiber	15	47
Sodium (mg)	2889	894
Vitamin C (mg)	42	607
B_1, thiamine (mg)	.8	2.1
B_6, pyridoxine (mg)	1.4	3.8
Iron (mg)	9.0	21
Folate (ug)	255	717
Magnesium (mg)	215	632
Calcium	746	735
Zinc (mg)	7.7	12.4
Selenium (ug)	59	88
Alpha tocopherol (mg)	4.9	5.5
Beta-carotene (ug)	786	26,302
Alpha-carotene (ug)	253	4420
Lutein & zeaxanthin (ug)	1257	64,055
Lycopene (ug)	795	2373
Total Nutrient Score	*19*	*85*

Menu III Comparison
Standard American Diet vs. Eat For Health Diet

Standard American Diet

Breakfast
- Bagel w/ cream cheese
- Orange juice

Lunch
- Bacon ranch salad w/ crispy chicken
- Ice tea

Dinner
- Chicken noodle soup
- Grilled cheese sandwich
- Potato salad
- Brownie

Eat For Health Diet

Breakfast
- Lettuce, Banana & Cashew Wrap*
- Pomegranate juice

Lunch
- Romaine & spinach salad w/ Creamy Blueberry Dressing*
- Fresh fruit & nut bowl

Dinner
- Raw veggies w/ Black Bean Dip*
- Dr. Fuhrman's Famous Anti-Cancer Soup*
- Yummy, Quick & Easy Banana Oat Bars*

See Menu III Nutrient Analysis on the next page.

* See recipes in Chapter 5, beginning on p. 63.

Menu III Nutritional Analysis
Standard American Diet vs. Eat For Health Diet

	SAD	EFH
Calories	2026	1985
Protein	67	70
Carbohydrate	212	335
Fat	105	56
Cholesterol (mg)	283	.25
Saturated fat	32	10
Fiber	11	62
Sodium (mg)	6832	1123
Vitamin C (mg)	167	495
B_1, thiamine (mg)	1.4	1.9
B_6, pyridoxine (mg)	.55	3.1
Iron (mg)	12.2	23
Folate (ug)	474	916
Magnesium (mg)	129	642
Calcium	625	824
Zinc (mg)	5.2	10.2
Selenium (ug)	62	129
Alpha tocopherol (mg)	2.9	9.7
Beta-carotene (ug)	1557	36,165
Alpha-carotene (ug)	17	6089
Lutein & zeaxanthin (ug)	385	64,395
Lycopene (ug)	0	3167
Total Nutrient Score	*19*	*91*

Chapter Five

High-Nutrient Recipes

H igh-nutrient recipes taste great and are good for you! Those that follow are among the most healthful recipes in the world. Enjoy them, create variations, and start on the road to your optimal weight and health.

Breakfasts

Blueberry Orange Smoothie
　1 cup frozen blueberries
　3 dates, pitted
　2 oranges, peeled
　1 banana
　1 Tbsp. ground flaxseed

Blend in blender until smooth.
Serves: 2

Lettuce, Banana & Cashew Wrap

2 tsp. Dr. Fuhrman's Raw Cashew Butter, per leaf
12 romaine lettuce leaves
2 bananas, thinly sliced

Spread cashew butter on lettuce leaf, lay banana slices on cashew butter, and wrap lettuce around. A delicious and healthful treat!

Serves: 2

Fruit & Nut Plate

1 cup blueberries
1 cup strawberries, sliced
1/2 green apple, sliced
8 walnuts, chopped

Place fruit on a plate and sprinkle with walnuts.

Serves: 1

Note: This recipe is just an example to give you an idea of the quantities you should use when making a dish like this. Feel free to use any variety of fruit and nuts.

Yummy, Quick & Easy Banana Oat Bars
2 cups quick oats (not instant)
1/4 cup chopped walnuts
1/2 cup shredded coconut
1/2 cup raisins or chopped dates
2 large ripe bananas, mashed
1/4 cup unsweetened applesauce, optional
1 Tbsp. date sugar, optional

Preheat oven to 350 degrees. Mix ingredients together in a large bowl. Press dough in a 9x9 inch baking pan. Bake for 30 minutes. Cool on wire rack. When cool, slice into squares or bars and serve.

If you'd like a sweeter, moister version of these bars, add the applesauce and date sugar.

Serves: 8

Soups

Dr. Fuhrman's Famous Anti-Cancer Soup

1 cup dried split peas and/or beans
4 cups water
4 medium onions
6-10 medium zucchini
3 leek stalks
2 bunches kale, collards, or other greens, chopped
  (stems and center ribs cut off and discarded)
4-5 cups fresh carrot juice
2 cups fresh organic celery juice
2 Tbsp. Dr. Fuhrman's VegiZest or other no-salt seasoning
1 cup raw cashews
8 oz. mushrooms (shiitake, cremini, or oyster), chopped

Set cashews and mushrooms aside. Put all other ingredients into a very large pot. Cover and simmer over low heat until onions, zucchini and leeks are soft (about 20 minutes). Remove the onions, zucchini, and leeks from the pot along with some of the soup liquid, being careful to leave the beans and some of the kale in the pot. Blend/puree the onions, zucchini, and leeks in a high-powered blender or food processor. Add more soup liquid and the cashews to the mixture and blend/puree. Return the blended, creamy mixture back to the pot. Add the mushrooms and simmer another 30 minutes, or until beans are soft.

Serves 6-8

Fast Black Bean Soup

2 15-oz. cans no-salt (or low-salt) black beans
2 cups frozen mixed vegetables
2 cups frozen corn
2 cups frozen chopped broccoli florets
2 cups fresh carrot juice
1 cup water
1 cup prepared no-salt or low-salt black bean soup
1/4 cup chopped cilantro (optional)
1/8 tsp. chili powder, or to taste
1 cup chopped fresh tomatoes
1 avocado, chopped or mashed
1/2 cup chopped green onions
1/4 cup raw pumpkin seeds (lightly toasted, if you like)

Combine first 9 ingredients in a soup pot. Bring to a boil and simmer on low heat for 30 minutes. Stir in fresh tomatoes and heat through. Serve topped with avocado, green onions, and pumpkin seeds.

Serves 5

Hearty Ginger Lentil Soup

8 cups fresh carrot juice
4 cups water
1 cup dried lentils
1/2 cup uncooked brown rice
2 zucchini, finely chopped
2 carrots, chopped
1 red bell pepper, finely chopped
1 onion, finely chopped
6 cloves garlic, minced or pressed
3 Tbsp. grated fresh ginger root
3 Tbsp. Dr. Fuhrman's VegiZest
1 tsp. ground coriander
1/2 tsp. ground cumin
1/8 tsp. ground allspice
2 sweet potatoes, peeled and cut into 1 inch cubes
2 bunches Swiss chard leaves and stems, chopped
1/2 cup chopped fresh parsley

In order listed, place all ingredients—except for the sweet potatoes, Swiss chard, and parsley—in a soup pot. Bring to a boil, cover, and simmer for 40 minutes. Add the potatoes, and simmer for another 15 minutes. Add the chard, and simmer for another 10 minutes. Serve topped with chopped parsley.

Serves 5

Salad Dressings

Russian Fig Dressing

4 Tbsp. no-salt or low-salt pasta sauce
3 Tbsp. Dr. Fuhrman's Almond Butter
2 Tbsp. Dr. Fuhrman's Black Fig Vinegar

Mash all ingredients together with a fork until smooth.
Serves 2

Orange Cashew Dressing

2 oranges, peeled and quartered
1/2 cup raw cashews (or 1/4 cup raw cashew butter)
2 Tbsp. Dr. Fuhrman's Blood Orange Vinegar
1/2 tsp. lemon juice (optional)

Blend all ingredients in a high-powered blender until smooth
and creamy (add orange juice if mixture gets too thick).
Yield: 1-1/2 cups

Creamy Blueberry Dressing

2 cups fresh (or frozen and thawed) blueberries
1/2 cup pomegranate juice
4 Tbsp. raw cashew butter
2 Tbsp. balsamic vinegar
1 Tbsp. Dr. Fuhrman's Spicy Pecan Vinegar

Blend all ingredients in a high-powered blender until smooth
and creamy.
Serves 4

Main Dishes

Chicken Dijon

2 boneless and skinless chicken breasts
4 Tbsp. fresh lime juice
2 cloves garlic, minced
2 Tbsp. vegan Worcestershire sauce
4 tsp. Dijon mustard

Trim all fat from chicken breasts. Mix lime juice, garlic, Worcestershire sauce, and Dijon mustard into a marinade. Put half the mixture aside and pour the rest over chicken. Marinate for 1/2 hour. Broil on low or grill for 7 minutes per side or until thoroughly cooked. Serve with rest of marinade spooned over top.

Serves: 2

Note: This is not a high-nutrient recipe, but it is much better than fried chicken, and it is a step in a healthier direction.

Vegetable Bean Burritos

1 head broccoli florets, chopped
1/2 head cauliflower florets, chopped
2 carrots, chopped
2 red peppers, chopped
1 zucchini, chopped
1 medium onion, chopped
1 tsp. basil

1 tsp. oregano
1 tsp. parsley
1 tsp. cumin
1/2 tsp. red pepper flakes or more, to taste
1 tsp. allspice (optional)
1-1/2 Tbsp. Dr. Fuhrman's VegiZest or other
  no-salt seasoning
4 cloves garlic
1 cup cashews
1/2 cup unsweetened soy milk
1 15-oz. can pinto beans (no salt added), drained

Topping
1/2 cup low-sodium pasta sauce, optional
1/2 cup shredded soy mozzarella cheese, optional

Wraps
8 whole wheat tortilla wraps or large romaine lettuce
leaves

Chop vegetables into small pieces by hand or in a food processor. In a large covered pot, sauté vegetables with herbs and spices in 1/8 cup water for 15 minutes or until tender. In the meantime, place cashews in food processor and chop until very fine. Add soy milk to the chopped cashews and blend until smooth. Add cashew/soy milk mixture and beans to the veggies and mix thoroughly. Spread mixture on tortilla or lettuce leaf and roll up to form burrito. Top with pasta sauce and shredded soy mozzarella cheese if desired.

Serves: 8

Pasta with Roasted Vegetables, Tomatoes & Basil

  2 red bell peppers, cut into 1/2 inch pieces
  1 medium eggplant, unpeeled, cut into 1/2 inch pieces
  1 large yellow crookneck squash, cut into 1/2 inch pieces
  1-1/2 cup butternut squash, peeled, cut into 1/2 inch
    pieces
  2 Tbsp. olive oil, divided
  1 lb. penne pasta, preferably whole wheat
  2 medium tomatoes, cored, seeded, diced
  1/2 cup chopped fresh basil or 1-1/2 Tbsp. dried
  2 Tbsp. balsamic vinegar or 1 Tbsp. fresh lemon juice
  2 cloves garlic, minced

Preheat oven to 450 degrees. Lightly coat roasting pan with 1/2 tsp. olive oil. Combine red bell peppers, eggplant, yellow squash, and butternut squash in prepared pan. Drizzle with 1 Tbsp. olive oil and toss to coat. Roast until vegetables are tender and beginning to brown, stirring occasionally, about 25 minutes.

Meanwhile, cook pasta and drain, reserving 1/2 cup cooking liquid.

Combine pasta, roasted vegetables, tomatoes, and basil in large bowl. Add remaining tablespoon of oil, vinegar, and garlic. Toss to combine. Add cooking liquid by tablespoon to moisten, if desired.

Serves: 6

Side Dishes

California Creamed Kale

2 bunches kale (bottoms of stems removed and discarded)
1 cup raw cashews
1 cup unsweetened soy milk
4 Tbsp. onion flakes
1 Tbsp. Dr. Fuhrman's VegiZest or other no-salt seasoning

Place kale leaves in a large steamer pot. Steam 10-20 minutes until soft. While kale is steaming, place remaining ingredients in a blender and blend until smooth. Place kale in colander, and press with a clean dish towel to remove some of the excess water. In a bowl, coarsely chop and mix kale with the cream sauce.

Serves 4

Note: Sauce may be used with broccoli, spinach, or other steamed veggies.

Baked Sweet Potato Fries

4 sweet potatoes
1 Tbsp. garlic powder
1 Tbsp. onion powder

Preheat oven to 400 degrees. Peel sweet potatoes if not organic. Cut into strips. Lay on a non-stick cookie sheet. Sprinkle garlic powder and onion powder on potatoes. Bake approximately 1-1/2 hours, turning potatoes every 15 minutes.

Serves 4

Tasty Hummus with Baked Garlic Pita Chips and Raw Veggies

Tasty Hummus:

1 cup cooked or canned garbanzo beans (no-salt or
  low-salt), reserving liquid
1/4 cup bean liquid or water
1/4 cup raw tahini (pureed sesame seeds)
1 Tbsp. lemon juice
1 Tbsp. Dr. Fuhrman's VegiZest or other no-salt seasoning
1 tsp. Bragg Liquid Aminos
1 tsp. horseradish (optional)
1 small clove garlic, chopped

Blend all ingredients in blender until creamy smooth. Use as
a spread or a dip for raw and lightly steamed vegetables.
Yield: 1 cup

Baked Garlic Pita Chips:

2 whole wheat pitas
Olive oil cooking spray (optional)
Garlic powder

Preheat oven to 375 degrees. Split each pita in half horizon-
tally. Spray pita halves lightly with olive oil, if desired, and
sprinkle with garlic powder. Cut each half in half and then
into four sections to form triangles. Place on baking sheet
and bake for 8 minutes or until lightly browned & crispy.
Serve with salsa or hummus.
Serves 2

Black Bean Dip

1 15 oz. can no-salt (or low-salt) black beans, drained
1 garlic clove
1/4 tsp. black pepper
1/8 tsp. chili pepper flakes
2 tsp. Dr. Fuhrman's VegiZest or other
  no-salt seasoning

Combine all ingredients in food processor with an S blade. Whirl to desired consistency, adding water one tablespoon at a time until desired consistency.

Serves: 2

Broccoli Vinaigrette

1 large bunch broccoli
1/4 cup seasoned rice vinegar
1 Tbsp. Dr. Fuhrman's VegiZest or other no-salt seasoning
2 tsp. Dijon mustard
2 large cloves garlic, pressed or minced

Break the broccoli into bite-sized florets. Peel stems and slice them into 1/4-inch-thick strips. Steam florets and stems for 8 minutes, or until just tender. While the broccoli is steaming, whisk the rest of the ingredients in bowl. Add broccoli and toss to mix.

Serves 2

Saucy Collards and Carrots

4 bunches collard greens (stems removed and discarded),
  chopped
4 carrots, grated
1/2 cup currants
Sauce:
1 medium cucumber
1/2 cup raisins
1/4 cup raw almond butter
2 tsp. Dr. Fuhrman's Riesling Raisin Vinegar (optional)
1 tsp. nutritional yeast

Set currants aside. Steam collard greens for 15 minutes. Add
grated carrots and steam another 5 minutes. Blend all sauce
ingredients in a high-powered blender until smooth. Add
currants and sauce to collards/carrots mixture and toss.
Serves 4

Desserts

Mango Coconut Sorbet

1/2 cup unsweetened shredded coconut
1/8 cup water
1/4 tsp. lemon or lime juice
1 10-oz. bag frozen mangos
3 slices dried mango, unsweetened and unsulfured

Reserve 1 Tbsp. coconut for garnish. Blend rest of ingredients in a high-powered blender. Garnish with reserved coconut.
Serves 4

Creamy Banana Fig Ice Cream

5 dried figs, stems removed
4 frozen bananas
5 Tbsp. unsweetened soy milk
2 tsp. Dr. Fuhrman's Black Fig Vinegar (optional)

Blend all ingredients in a high-powered blender until creamy.
Serves 4

Note: To freeze ripe bananas: Peel, cut in thirds, wrap tightly in plastic wrap, and freeze at least 24 hrs. before making recipe.

Dr. Fuhrman's Wild Apple Crunch

6 apples, peeled and sliced
3/4 cup chopped walnuts
8 dates, chopped
1 cup currants or raisins
3/4 cup water
1/2 tsp. cinnamon
1/4 tsp. nutmeg
Juice of 1 orange

Preheat oven to 375 degrees. Combine all ingredients except the orange juice. Place in a baking pan and sprinkle the juice of the orange on top. Cover and bake at 375 degrees for about one hour until all ingredients are soft, stirring occasionally.
Serves 8

Note: You also can simmer this for 30 minutes on top of the stove in a covered pot, stirring occasionally.

Chapter Six

Your Commitment to Health

My goal in writing this book is to help you say "no" to our culture of disease and drugs and to say "yes" to lifelong health and happiness. If an army of Americans made the few simple, but profound, dietary and lifestyle changes I recommend, we quickly would win the war against heart disease, diabetes, strokes, and cancers.

By following the recommendations in this book, virtually everyone can improve their health, and if you start in time, you actually can make yourself heart-attack proof. I believe all people should be informed that they have this opportunity to protect themselves. There is no magic to it. Educating yourself with the latest scientific findings and eating a diet of delicious, high-nutrient food allows you to protect yourself and your family from the health tragedies you see all around you—and not just the big tragedies like heart disease. Allergies, joint pain, fatigue, headaches, mental clarity, and digestive problems *all* can dramatically resolve through nutritional excellence.

Those who truly desire to protect themselves can do so, without expensive and risky prescription drugs. Proper self-care is more effective and overwhelmingly less expensive than conventional care.

It is not an exaggeration to say that you are in a fight for your life. Don't let food manufacturers and fast food establishments take your health away. Fight back against junk food and food addiction.

Good information is the most powerful artillery you have to save your life and the lives of loved ones. Be a fighter. Learn and encourage others. Working together, we can change the nutritional landscape of America, save lives, and save our economy that is slowly being destroyed by out-of-control healthcare costs. Join the growing army of Americans who are choosing nutritional excellence, and reclaim your right to a long life of health and happiness.

Getting started

This book will get you started in the right direction, but if you want more information and are ready to take it to the next level, visit www.EatRightAmerica.com or call (877) ERA-4-USA to get my comprehensive two-book set, *Eat For Health*. The complete *Eat For Health* approach offers you motivational tools, menu plans, and great tasting recipes for superior health. It also teaches you the science behind nutritional excellence. This four-step body makeover and disease-reversal program will help you overcome your addictions and achieve your ideal weight and health.

High-nutrient eating

The pages that follow show you the nutrient density scores of virtually all of the categories of foods typically eaten in America. First is the list of my Top 30 Super Foods—the most wholesome foods with the highest nutrient ratings in the best categories. Then come the comprehensive lists of all of the foods by category. Use these scores regularly until you are confident that your diet is as nutrient-rich as it can be.

Chapter Seven

Dr. Fuhrman's Top 30 Super Foods

N ow that you know the secret formula to health is $H = N/C$ (health = nutrients/calories), it's time to start putting it into practice. There are comprehensive lists of nutrient density scores in the next chapter. But to make it easy for you to find the very best foods, I've listed my Top 30 Super Foods below. These are the best foods in the best categories. For weight loss and improved health, include as many of these foods in your diet as you possibly can.

	Dr. Fuhrman's *Top 30 Super Foods*	*Nutrient* *Score*
1.	Collard, mustard, & turnip greens	1000
2.	Kale	1000
3.	Watercress	1000
4.	Bok choy	824
5.	Spinach	739
6.	Brussels sprouts	672

7.	Swiss chard	670
8.	Arugula	559
9.	Radish	554
10.	Cabbage	481
11.	Bean sprouts	444
12.	Red peppers	420
13.	Romaine lettuce	389
14.	Broccoli	376
15.	Carrot juice	344
16.	Tomatoes & tomato products	190-300
17.	Cauliflower	295
18.	Strawberries	212
19.	Pomegranate juice	193
20.	Blackberries	178
21.	Plums	157
22.	Raspberries	145
23.	Blueberries	130
24.	Papaya	118
25.	Brazil nuts	116
26.	Oranges	109
27.	Tofu	86
28.	Beans (all varieties)	55-70
29.	Seeds: flaxseed, sunflower, sesame	45
30.	Walnuts	29

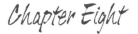
Chapter Eight

Nutrient Density Scores

In this chapter, you will find extensive lists of nutrient/calorie-density scores grouped by category based on my "Aggregate Nutrient Density Index"* (ANDI). Knowing which foods are high in nutrient density (and which are low) will make it easier to get the dramatic health benefits of eating more high-nutrient foods.

For optimal health, I suggest you consume an appropriate number of calories to meet your needs, keep your sodium intake below 1000 mg per day, and eat as many foods with high ANDI scores as possible.

ANDI Scores

ANDI scores are calculated by evaluating an extensive range of food factors, including vitamins, minerals, phytochemicals, and antioxidant capacities, based on an equal number of calories for each food. After completing the calculations,

* Patent Pending

foods are ranked on a numerical scale of 1 to 1000, with the highest nutrient foods given a score of 1000.

A complete description of how ANDI scores are calculated appears in my two-book set, *Eat For Health.* To order, visit www.EatRightAmerica.com or call (877) ERA-4-USA.

Easy-to-get benefits

While nutrient scores are calculated using sophisticated scientific considerations, you don't have to be a scientist to get the many benefits of high-nutrient food, recipes, and menus.

Simply take the information you've learned from this book, put it into practice, and start on the road to a thinner, healthier you—*today!*

| Food item
Description/portion size	Calories	Sodium	ANDI score

Beans/Legumes

Adzuki beans, boiled (1 cup)	294	18	56
Baked beans w/ pork, canned (1 cup)	268	1047	20
Baked beans w/ pork in tomato sauce, canned (1 cup)	238	1106	32
Black beans, boiled (1 cup)	227	2	58
Eden Foods Organic No Salt Added Black Beans (1 cup)	220	30	58
Black-eyed peas, boiled (1 cup)	198	7	67
Chickpeas, boiled (1 cup)	269	11	48
Chickpeas, canned (1 cup)	286	718	55
Chile con carne w/ beans, canned (222g)	269	941	21
Chili w/ beans, canned (1 cup)	287	1336	27
Edamame (1 cup)	254	25	58
Fava beans, boiled (1 cup)	187	8	61
Great Northern beans, boiled (1 cup)	209	4	61
Kidney beans, boiled (1 cup)	225	2	56
Kidney beans, canned (1 cup)	213	770	71
Westbrae Organic Kidney Beans (1 cup)	200	280	71
Lentils, boiled (1 cup)	230	4	68
Lima beans, boiled (1 cup)	216	4	60
Navy beans, boiled (1 cup)	255	0	57
Pinto beans, boiled (1 cup)	245	2	57
Refried beans, canned (1 cup)	238	756	59
Soybeans, boiled (1 cup)	298	2	48
Split peas, boiled (1 cup)	231	4	56
White beans, boiled (1 cup)	249	11	51

Beverages

Alcohol

Beer (12 fluid oz.)	139	14	7
Wine, red (4 fluid oz.)	80	6	3
Wine, white (4 fluid oz.)	80	6	3

Food item Description/portion size	Calo ries	Sod ium	ANDI score
Cocoa			
Hot cocoa, prepared w/ milk (8 fluid oz.)	192	110	18
Hot cocoa, prepared w/ water (8 fluid oz.)	113	146	10
Dairy			
Buttermilk, low-fat (8 fluid oz.)	98	257	25
Chocolate milk, low-fat (8 fluid oz.)	158	152	19
Chocolate milk, whole (8 fluid oz.)	207	150	14
Eggnog (8 fluid oz.)	343	137	11
Evaporated milk (2 Tbsp.)	42	33	14
Half & Half cream (2 Tbsp.)	39	12	8
Heavy whipping cream (2 Tbsp.)	104	11	2
Milk, low-fat 1% (8 fluid oz.)	105	127	28
Milk, non-fat skim (8 fluid oz.)	83	103	36
Milk, reduced-fat 2% (8 fluid oz.)	122	100	23
Milk, whole 3.3% (8 fluid oz.)	146	98	20
Milk shake, chocolate (8 fluid oz.)	270	252	11
Milk shake, vanilla (8 fluid oz.)	254	215	11
Sweetened condensed milk (2 Tbsp.)	123	49	9
Fruit Drinks			
Capri Sun Juice Drink, Fruit Punch (210g)	99	21	1
Fruit punch, added vitamin C (8 fluid oz.)	117	94	30*
Fruit punch, no added nutrients (8 fluid oz.)	109	23	4
Kool Aid Burst, Tropical Punch (210g)	90	29	0
Lemonade, from dry mix (8 fluid oz.)	103	11	6
Lemonade, from frozen concentrate (8 fluid oz.)	131	7	7
Juices			
Apple juice, unsweetened (8 fluid oz.)	117	7	16
Apricot nectar (8 fluid oz.)	141	8	23
Carrot, bottled (8 fluid oz.)	98	71	344

* Artificially inflated nutrient score due to fortification with vitamins and minerals.

Food item Description/portion size	Calories	Sodium	ANDI score
Cranberry juice cocktail (8 fluid oz.)	144	5	55
Grape (8 fluid oz.)	150	25	20*
Grapefruit, unsweetened (8 fluid oz.)	101	2	74
Orange (8 fluid oz.)	112	2	86
Pineapple (8 fluid oz.)	140	2	33
Pomegranate juice (8 fluid oz.)	150	10	193
Tomato (8 fluid oz.)	41	656	342
Tomato, low-sodium (8 fluid oz.)	41	24	342
Vegetable, low-sodium (8 fluid oz.)	46	140	365
Vegetable, regular (8 fluid oz.)	46	653	365

Non-Dairy Milk

Almond milk (8 fluid oz.)	211	14	19
Rice milk (8 fluid oz.)	120	86	10
Soy milk (8 fluid oz.)	125	132	33

Soda

Cola (8 fluid oz.)	119	11	1
Diet cola (8 fluid oz.)	0	38	0
Diet Sprite (8 fluid oz.)	0	14	0
Root beer (8 fluid oz.)	101	32	1
Seltzer (8 fluid oz.)	0	50	0
Sprite (8 fluid oz.)	98	27	1
Tonic water (8 fluid oz.)	83	10	1

Sports Drinks

Flavored sports drink (8 fluid oz.)	60	96	1

Artificially inflated nutrient score due to fortification with vitamins and minerals.

Food item *Description/portion size*	Calo ries	Sod ium	ANDI score

Bread/Grain Products

Bagels
Bagel, plain (1 bagel)	195	379	18*
Bagel, whole-grain (1 bagel)	181	360	18*

Biscuits
Biscuit, plain (1 biscuit)	212	348	11*

Bread
Bread, sprouted-grain (Manna type) 1 slice (56g)	130	3	39
Bread, 100% whole wheat (2 slices)	130	265	25
Bread, white (2 slices)	133	340	18*
Bread crumbs, commercially prepared (1/4 cup)	107	198	18*
Bread sticks, commercially prepared (2 bread sticks)	82	131	15*
Dinner roll, whole wheat (2 rolls)	151	272	22
Dinner roll, plain, ready to eat (2 rolls)	170	296	16*
French (2 slices)	137	304	19*
Hamburger roll (1 roll)	120	206	17*
Hard roll (1 roll)	167	310	18*
Hot dog roll (1 roll)	120	206	17*
Italian (2 slices)	163	350	19*
Mixed grain (2 slices)	130	253	30
Mixed grain hamburger roll (1 roll)	113	197	21
Pita, plain (1 pita)	165	322	18*
Pita, whole wheat (1 pita)	170	340	19
Pumpernickel (2 slices)	160	429	19*
Raisin (2 slices)	142	203	16*
Rye (2 slices)	166	422	20*

* Artificially inflated nutrient score due to fortification with vitamins and minerals.

Food item Description/portion size	Calo ries	Sod ium	ANDI score
Crackers			
Cheese cracker sandwich w/ cheese (4 crackers)	127	228	10*
Cheese cracker sandwich w/ peanut butter (4 crackers)	139	199	10*
Cheese crackers (30 crackers)	151	298	13*
Graham crackers (2-1/2" sq.) (4 crackers)	118	169	8*
Health Valley Amaranth Graham Cracker (8 crackers)	100	30	11*
Health Valley Low-Fat Whole Wheat Cracker (6 crackers)	60	140	15
Kashi TLC Original 7 Grain Cracker (15 crackers)	130	160	13
Low-salt whole wheat crackers (7 crackers)	124	69	14
Matzo crackers (1 cracker)	112	1	11*
Melba toast (3 slices)	58	124	15*
Melba toast, unsalted (3 slices)	58	3	12*
Nabisco Ritz Crackers (5 crackers) (16g)	79	124	7*
Nabisco Snackwell's Wheat Crackers (5 crackers) (15g)	62	150	10*
Nabisco Snackwell's Zesty Cheese Crackers (1.1 oz.) (30g)	129	315	7*
Nabisco Wheat Thins Crackers (16 crackers) (29g)	136	168	7*
Rice cake cracker (7 crackers)	115	21	12
Rye crispbread (Finn Crisp or Wasa brands) (1 cracker)	37	26	20
Saltines (5 crackers)	64	161	11*
Saltines, low-salt (5 crackers)	65	95	13*
Soda crackers (5 crackers)	64	161	11*
Triscuit wafers (7 crackers)	140	230	17
English Muffins			
English muffin, enriched (1 muffin)	134	264	13*
English muffin, whole wheat (1 muffin)	134	420	28
French toast, frozen (2 slices)	251	584	22*
Grains			
Amaranth (1 cup, cooked)	240	13	23
Barley, pearled (1 cup, cooked)	193	5	32
Cornmeal, whole grain (1 cup, cooked)	143	5	22

Artificially inflated nutrient score due to fortification with vitamins and minerals.

Food item Description/portion size	Calories	Sodium	ANDI score
Couscous, (1 cup, cooked)	176	8	15
Millet (1 cup, cooked)	250	3	19
Quinoa (1 cup, cooked)	210	12	21
Rice, brown (1 cup, cooked)	216	10	41
Rice, white (1 cup, cooked)	205	2	12*
Rice, white w/ pasta, (Rice a Roni type) (1 cup, cooked)	246	1147	15*
Rice, wild brown (1 cup, cooked)	166	5	43

Matzo

Matzo, commercially prepared (1 sheet)	111	6	13*
Matzo, crackers (1 cracker)	112	1	11*

Muffins/Quick Bread

Banana bread (1 slice)	196	181	8*
Blueberry (1 muffin)	158	255	10*
Bran (1 muffin)	161	335	19*
Corn (1 muffin)	174	297	13*

Pancakes

Pancakes, frozen (3 pancakes)	247	550	17*
Kelloggs Eggo Buttermilk Pancakes (3 pancakes)	270	615	14*
Pancakes, prepared (3 pancakes)	259	500	13*

Pasta

Macaroni & cheese, canned (209g)	171	880	16
Pasta, cooked (2 cups)	395	3	18*
Pasta, spinach, cooked (2 cups)	333	15	15
Pasta, whole wheat, cooked (2 cups)	347	8	19
Pasta, w/ meatballs, in tomato sauce, canned (250g)	258	1045	18
Tortellini (1-1/2 cups)	497	557	13*

* Artificially inflated nutrient score due to fortification with vitamins and minerals.

Food item Description/portion size	Calo ries	Sod ium	ANDI score
Stuffing			
Bread stuffing, mix, prepared (1/2 cup)	178	543	20*
Tacos			
Taco shell (2 tacos)	124	98	11*
Tortillas			
Corn (2 tortillas)	113	23	12*
Flour (2 tortillas)	200	407	15*
Waffles (frozen)			
Plain waffle, frozen (2 waffles)	176	524	28*
Kelloggs Eggo Lowfat Blueberry Nutri Grain (2 waffles)	146	414	24*
Kellogg's Eggo Lowfat Homestyle (2 waffles)	165	309	28*

Cereals

Cold Cereals			
Amaranth flakes (1 cup)	134	14	20
Chocolate flavored rings, presweetened (1 cup)	150	171	42*
Cocoa rice cereal (1 cup)	122	203	68*
Corn flakes cereal, sweetened (1 cup)	149	247	42*
Crisp rice cereal (1 cup)	111	206	46*
Frosted oat cereal w/ marshmallows (1 cup)	109	158	54*
Granola cereal, prepared (1 cup)	598	27	22
Puffed rice cereal, fortified (1 cup)	57	1	42*
Puffed wheat cereal, fortified (1 cup)	44	1	61*
Shredded wheat, large biscuit (2 biscuits)	159	3	26
Hot Cereals			
Cream of rice (1 cup)	127	3	6
Cream of wheat (1 cup)	149	9	82*

Artificially inflated nutrient score due to fortification with vitamins and minerals.

Food item Description/portion size	Calo ries	Sod ium	ANDI score
Farina cereal (1 cup)	94	109	66*
Instant oatmeal w/raisins & spice, fortified (1 package)	158	248	74*
Oats, cooked w/ water (1 cup)	147	2	53
Roman meal w/ oats (1 cup)	171	9	51

Cereals *(by brand)*

Alpen Cereal
Alpen Cereal (1 cup)	398	240	22

Familia Cereal
Familia Cereal (1 cup)	474	61	22

General Mills
Basic 4 (1 cup)	202	316	32*
Cheerios (1 cup)	111	214	84*
Chex (1 cup)	112	288	62*
Cinnamon Toast Crunch (1 cup)	169	275	45*
Cocoa Puffs (1 cup)	117	172	49*
Fiber One (1 cup)	118	258	135*
Honey Nut Cheerios (1 cup)	112	270	61*
Kix (1 cup)	85	201	67*
Lucky Charms (1 cup)	114	204	58*
Reese's Puffs (1 cup)	170	222	45*
Total (1 cup)	84	158	249*
Trix (1 cup)	118	194	49*
Wheaties (1 cup)	107	218	106*

Kashi
Go Lean (1 cup)	148	86	28
Good Friends (1 cup)	168	130	27
Heart to Heart (1 cup)	147	120	129*

* Artificially inflated nutrient score due to fortification with vitamins and minerals.

Food item Description/portion size	Calo ries	Sod ium	ANDI score
Kelloggs			
All-Bran (1 cup)	115	285	236*
Apple Jacks (1 cup)	129	157	46*
Complete Oat Bran Flakes (1 cup)	140	280	257*
Corn Flakes (1 cup)	101	203	75*
Corn Pops (1 cup)	118	120	39*
Frosted Flakes (1 cup)	152	198	43*
Frosted Mini-Wheats (1 cup)	174	5	47*
Fruit Loops (1 cup)	118	151	71*
Meuslix (1 cup)	293	254	70*
Rice Krispies (1 cup)	95	255	62*
Shredded Wheat (1 cup)	103	5	64*
Smart Start (1 cup)	182	275	136*
Special K (1 cup)	118	224	118*
Post			
100% Bran (1 cup)	252	367	82*
Cocoa Pebbles (1 cup)	154	209	38*
Frosted Alpha-Bits (1 cup)	130	212	36*
Grape Nuts (1 cup)	417	708	39*
Honey Bunches of Oats (1 cup)	158	257	44*
Quaker			
Quaker Corn Grits, instant (137g)	93	288	29*
Quaker Instant Oatmeal w/Apples & Cinnamon (149g)	130	165	57*
Quaker Instant Oatmeal w/Raisins, Dates & Walnuts (100g)	116	207	48*
Cap'n Crunch (1 cup)	145	270	66*
Oatmeal Squares (1 cup)	212	269	48*
Quaker Oat Cinnamon Life (1 cup)	160	204	68*
Ralston			
Ralston Cereal (1 cup)	134	476	60

* Artificially inflated nutrient score due to fortification with vitamins and minerals.

Food item Description/portion size	Calories	Sodium	ANDI score
Wheatena			
Wheatena (1 cup)	136	5	52*

Dairy Products & Eggs

Cheese

American (2 oz.)	213	369	10
Blue cheese (2 oz.)	200	791	12
Brie cheese (2 oz.)	189	357	12
Cheddar cheese (2 oz.)	229	352	11
Cheddar, low-fat (2 oz.)	98	347	16
Cottage cheese (1 cup)	216	850	13
Cottage cheese, low-fat (1 cup)	163	918	18
Cream cheese (4 Tbsp.)	202	172	4
Cream cheese, fat-free (4 Tbsp.)	58	327	18
Feta cheese (2 oz.)	150	633	21
Goat cheese (2 oz.)	206	292	8
Gruyere cheese (2 oz.)	234	191	13
Monterey Jack cheese (2 oz.)	211	304	12
Mozzarella cheese, non-fat (2 oz.)	84	420	35
Mozzarella cheese, part skim (2 oz.)	144	351	16
Mozzarella cheese, whole milk (2 oz.)	170	356	14
Muenster cheese (2 oz.)	209	356	12
Parmesan (2 Tbsp.)	43	153	15
Ricotta cheese, part skim (1/2 cup)	170	154	16
Ricotta, whole milk (1/2 cup)	214	103	11
Swiss cheese (2 oz.)	215	109	15
Swiss cheese, low-fat (2 oz.)	101	147	29
Swiss cheese, low-sodium (2 slices)	213	8	14

* Artificially inflated nutrient score due to fortification with vitamins and minerals.

| Food item
Description/portion size | Calo
ries | Sod
ium | ANDI
score |
|---|---|---|---|
| **Cream Products** | | | |
| Reddi Whip Fat-Free Whipped Topping (3 oz.) | 127 | 61 | 17 |
| Sour cream (2 Tbsp.) | 51 | 13 | 5 |
| Sour cream, fat-free (2 Tbsp.) | 24 | 45 | 16 |
| Sour cream, light (2 Tbsp.) | 33 | 17 | 9 |
| Sour cream, non-fat (2 Tbsp.) | 24 | 45 | 16 |
| Sour cream, reduced fat (2 Tbsp.) | 54 | 21 | 8 |
| **Eggs** | | | |
| Egg (1 egg) | 74 | 70 | 27 |
| Egg substitute, liquid (1/2 cup) | 106 | 222 | 31 |
| Egg substitute, powder (1 oz.) | 126 | 227 | 27 |
| Egg white (1 egg white) | 17 | 55 | 30 |
| Egg yolk (1 egg yolk) | 53 | 8 | 23 |
| **Yogurt** | | | |
| Fruit yogurt, low-fat (1 cup) | 250 | 142 | 14 |
| Fruit yogurt, non-fat (1 cup) | 230 | 142 | 16 |
| Plain yogurt, low-fat (1 cup) | 154 | 172 | 26 |
| Plain yogurt, non-fat (1 cup) | 137 | 189 | 32 |
| Plain yogurt, whole milk (1 cup) | 149 | 113 | 18 |
| Vanilla yogurt, low-fat (1 cup) | 208 | 162 | 19 |
| Vanilla yogurt, non-fat (1 cup) | 98 | 134 | 30 |

Desserts

Cakes			
Angel food cake, ready to eat (1 slice)	73	213	9 *
Butter pound cake, ready to eat (1 slice)	291	298	5 *
Carrot cake w/ cream cheese frosting (1 slice)	484	273	4 *
Cheesecake, ready to eat (1 slice)	385	248	4 *
Chocolate cake w/ frosting (1 slice)	235	214	5 *

* Artificially inflated nutrient score due to fortification with vitamins and minerals.

Food item Description/portion size	Calo ries	Sod ium	ANDI score
Chocolate cake, prepared (1 slice)	340	299	7*
Chocolate snack cake, creme filled w/frosting (1 cake)	188	212	8*
Chocolate snack cake, low-fat w/ frosting (1 cake)	131	178	5*
Cinnamon coffee cake w/ crumb topping (1 slice)	237	199	8*
Devil's food cake w/ chocolate frosting (1 slice)	235	214	5*
Fruitcake, ready to eat (1 piece)	139	116	5*
Pound cake, fat-free, ready to eat (1 slice)	160	193	6*
Shortcake, biscuit type, prepared (1 biscuit)	225	329	9*
Sponge cake, ready to eat (1 slice)	110	93	9*
Yellow cake w/frosting (1 slice)	239	220	3*

Pastry & Pie

Apple pie, prepared (1 slice)	411	327	6*
Blueberry pie, prepared (1 slice)	360	272	5*
Boston cream pie, prepared (1 slice)	398	355	9*
Butter croissant (1 croissant)	231	424	9*
Cheese croissant (1 croissant)	236	316	11*
Cinnamon Danish pastry (1 pastry)	262	241	5*
Cinnamon sweet roll w/ frosting (1 roll)	223	230	11*
Pecan pie, prepared (1 slice)	452	479	5*
Pumpkin pie, prepared (1 slice)	316	349	18*

Desserts *(Frozen)*

Frozen Bars

Frozen fruit & juice bar (1 bar)	75	4	9
Ice pop or Popsicle (1 pop)	42	7	0
Sundae ice cream novelty (2 oz.)	105	54	8

Frozen Yogurt

Chocolate frozen yogurt (1 cup)	221	110	13
Vanilla frozen yogurt (1 cup)	235	125	9

* Artificially inflated nutrient score due to fortification with vitamins and minerals.

Food item *Description/portion size*	*Calo ries*	*Sod ium*	*ANDI score*
Ice Cream			
Chocolate ice cream (1 cup)	377	84	6
Chocolate ice cream, light (1 cup) (136g)	271	97	6
Hot fudge sundae (1 sundae)	284	182	9
Strawberry ice cream (1 cup)	253	79	9
Strawberry sundae (1 sundae)	268	92	8
Vanilla ice cream (1 cup)	289	115	9
Vanilla ice cream, light (1 cup)	218	98	10
Vanilla ice cream w/ cone, soft-serve (1 ice cream cone)	164	92	10
Ice Cream Cones (without ice cream)			
Ice cream cone, sugar (1 cone)	40	32	11
Ice cream cone, wafer (1 cone)	17	6	10
Sherbet			
Fruit ice, reduced-calorie (1 fruit ice)	12	3	3
Italian ice, restaurant-prepared (1 cup)	123	9	4
Pineapple coconut ice (1 cup)	217	67	11
Sherbet, all flavors (1 cup)	213	68	9

Dressings/Sauces/Dips/Spreads

Dressings			
Annie's Natural Lowfat Mustard Vinaigrette (3 Tbsp.)	68	300	3
Balsamic vinegar (2 Tbsp.)	4	0	17
Blue cheese (3 Tbsp.)	231	502	4
Blue cheese, low-calorie (3 Tbsp.)	45	540	8
Caesar (3 Tbsp.)	233	475	2
Maple Grove Farms Caesar (3 Tbsp.)	15	90	4
French (3 Tbsp.)	214	391	4
French, fat-free (3 Tbsp.)	63	384	4

Food item Description/portion size	Calories	Sodium	ANDI score
French, low-fat (3 Tbsp.)	113	393	8
Walden Farms Classic French (3 Tbsp.)	0	285	3
Italian (3 Tbsp.)	128	729	6
Italian, fat-free (3 Tbsp.)	20	474	18
Italian, reduced-calorie (3 Tbsp.)	84	597	2
Mayonnaise (2 Tbsp.)	115	209	2
Mayonnaise, low-calorie (2 Tbsp.)	76	200	3
Oil & vinegar dressing (3 Tbsp.)	210	0	3
Ranch (3 Tbsp.)	203	343	4
Ranch, fat-free (3 Tbsp.)	50	317	5
Ranch, reduced-fat (3 Tbsp.)	92	391	5
Russian (3 Tbsp.)	227	398	5

Oils

Canola oil (1 Tbsp.)	120	0	3
Corn oil (1 Tbsp.)	120	0	3
Olive oil (1 Tbsp.)	119	0	2
Peanut oil (1 Tbsp.)	119	0	2
Safflower oil (1 Tbsp.)	120	0	6
Sesame oil (1 Tbsp.)	120	0	1
Soybean oil (1 Tbsp.)	120	0	3
Sunflower oil (1 Tbsp.)	120	0	8

Sauces

Barbecue (2 Tbsp.)	23	255	19
Beef gravy, canned (1/4 cup)	31	325	12
Cheese (1/4 cup)	121	578	7
Chicken gravy, canned (1/4 cup)	47	346	7
Cranberry (1/4 cup)	105	20	3
Fish sauce (1 Tbsp.)	6	1390	88
Hoisin sauce (1 Tbsp.)	35	258	7
Horseradish, prepared (1 Tbsp.)	7	47	52

Food item Description/portion size	Calories	Sodium	ANDI score
Ketchup (1 Tbsp.)	15	166	91
Ketchup, low-sodium (1 Tbsp.)	16	3	92
Marinara sauce, canned (1/2 cup)	92	601	119
Mustard (1 tsp.)	3	56	47
Oyster sauce (1 Tbsp.)	8	437	20
Soy sauce (1 Tbsp.)	10	1029	30
Soy sauce, low-sodium (1 Tbsp.)	10	600	32
Teriyaki sauce (1 Tbsp.)	15	690	15
Tomato sauce, canned (1/4 cup)	20	321	248
Tomato sauce, canned, low-sodium (1/4 cup)	20	20	247
Walnut Acres Low-Sodium Tomato & Basil Sauce (1/2 cup)	40	20	119

Spreads/Dips

Butter (1 Tbsp.)	102	82	1
Chocolate hazelnut spread (2 Tbsp.)	173	13	7
Hummus (1/2 cup)	218	298	70
Jam or preserves (1 Tbsp.)	56	6	3
Jelly (1 Tbsp.)	51	6	1
Margarine (1 Tbsp.)	101	133	3
Margarine butter blend (1 Tbsp.)	102	127	2
Salsa (2 Tbsp.)	4	96	236
Tahini (2 Tbsp.)	178	10	30

Toppings

Caramel topping (2 Tbsp.)	103	143	2
Marshmallow topping (1 oz.)	91	23	0
Whipped cream topping, pressurized (2 Tbsp.)	19	10	3
Whipped topping, low-fat, frozen (1/2 cup)	82	27	3

Food item Description/portion size	Calo ries	Sod ium	ANDI score

Fast Foods

Breakfast

Biscuit w/ egg & bacon (1)	457	999	11*
Biscuit w/ egg & ham (1)	442	1382	16*
Biscuit w/ egg & sausage (1)	410	888	14*
Biscuit w/ egg, cheese & bacon (1)	477	1260	10*
Biscuit w/ ham (1)	386	1433	11*
Croissant w/ egg, cheese & bacon (1)	413	889	10*
Croissant w/ egg, cheese & ham (1)	474	1081	11*
Croissant w/ egg, cheese & sausage (1)	523	1115	10*
English muffin w/ cheese & sausage (1)	393	1036	13*
English muffin w/ egg, cheese & sausage (1)	487	1135	14*

Burgers

Cheeseburger, double patty w/condiments & vegetables (1)	417	1051	14*
Cheeseburger, double patty, plain (1)	457	635	15*
Cheeseburger, w/ condiments & vegetables (1)	359	976	14*
Composite fast-food hamburger/cheeseburger (1)	287	495	11*
Hamburger, plain (1)	274	387	14*
Hamburger, double patty, plain (1)	544	554	14*
Hamburger, double patty, w/condiments & vegetables (1)	576	742	14*
Hamburger, triple patty, large w/ condiments & pickles (1)	692	712	17*
McDonald's Big Mac (1)	495	737	16*
McDonald's Big Mac w/ cheese (1)	572	1062	16*
McDonald's Cheeseburger (1)	326	739	15*
McDonald's Hamburger (1)	270	502	16*
McDonald's Quarter Pounder (1)	438	640	17*
McDonald's Quarter Pounder w/ cheese (1)	535	1176	16*

Chicken

Chicken fillet sandwich w/ cheese (1)	632	1238	12*
Chicken fillet sandwich, plain (1)	515	957	11*

* Artificially inflated nutrient score due to fortification with vitamins and minerals.

Food item *Description/portion size*	Calo ries	Sod ium	*ANDI* *score*
McDonald's Chicken McGrill Sandwich (1)	422	1240	17*
McDonald's Crispy Chicken Sandwich (1)	537	1424	13*

Fish
Fish sandwich w/ tartar sauce & cheese (1)	523	939	15*
Fish sandwich w/ tartar sauce (1)	431	615	15*
McDonald's Filet-O-Fish Sandwich (1)	415	663	11*

Mexican
Burrito w/ beans & meat (2)	508	1335	16*
Burrito w/ beans, cheese & beef (2)	331	991	17*
Burrito w/ fruit (apple or cherry), fast food (1)	231	212	8*
Burrito w/ beans (2)	447	985	14*
Chili con carne (1 cup)	256	1007	26
Chimichanga w/ beef & cheese (1)	443	957	15*
Enchilada w/ beef & cheese (1)	323	1319	14*
Nachos (113g)	346	816	11*
Nachos w/ cheese & jalapeno peppers (204g)	608	1736	10*
Nachos w/ cinnamon & sugar (109g)	592	439	6*
Nachos w/cheese, beans, ground beef & peppers (255g)	569	1800	11*
Taco, prepared (1)	369	802	16*
Tostada w/ guacamole (1)	181	401	18*
Tostada w/ beans & cheese (1)	223	543	14*
Tostada w/ beef & cheese (1)	315	897	17*

Milk Shakes
Chocolate milk shake (8 fluid oz.)	211	161	12
Strawberry milk shake (8 fluid oz.)	256	188	10
Vanilla milk shake (8 fluid oz.)	184	136	11

* Artificially inflated nutrient score due to fortification with vitamins and minerals.

Food item *Description/portion size*	*Calo ries*	*Sod ium*	*ANDI score*
Pizza			
Cheese pizza (2 slices)	281	672	17*
Combination pizza, w/ meat & vegetables (2 slices)	368	765	15*
Pepperoni pizza (2 slices)	362	534	13*
Sandwiches			
Roast beef sandwich w/ cheese (1)	473	1633	16*
Roast beef sandwich, plain (1)	346	792	16*
Submarine w/ cold cuts, cheese & vegetables (1)	456	1651	18*
Submarine w/ roast beef, mayonnaise & vegetables (1)	410	845	16*
Submarine w/ tuna salad (1)	584	1293	14*
Side Orders			
Coleslaw (1 cup)	195	356	8
French fried potatoes, fried in vegetable oil (2-1/2 oz.)	242	140	7
Hashed brown potatoes (1/2 cup)	151	290	7
McDonald's French Fries (medium bag)	412	195	7
Potato salad (1/2 cup)	164	472	9
Tossed Vegetable Salads			
Salad w/cheese & egg, no dressing (1-1/2 cups)	102	119	26
Salad w/chicken, no dressing (1-1/2 cups)	105	209	38
Salad w/pasta & seafood, no dressing (1-1/2 cups)	379	1572	21
Salad w/ shrimp, no dressing (1-1/2 cups)	106	489	50

* Artificially inflated nutrient score due to fortification with vitamins and minerals.

Food item Description/portion size	Calo ries	Sod ium	ANDI score

Fish

Canned

Food item	Calories	Sodium	ANDI score
Anchovies, canned in oil (4 anchovies)	34	587	43
Clams, drained (4 oz.)	168	127	338
Salmon (4 oz.)	158	628	42
Sardines, canned in oil (4 sardines)	100	242	42
Tuna, in oil (4 oz.)	211	449	32
Tuna, in water (4 oz.)	145	428	36

Fillets

Food item	Calories	Sodium	ANDI score
Bass, freshwater, cooked, dry heat (4 oz.)	166	102	22
Bluefish, cooked, dry heat (4 oz.)	180	87	41
Catfish, wild, cooked, dry heat (4 oz.)	119	57	29
Cod, cooked, dry heat (4 oz.)	119	88	31
Flounder, cooked, dry heat (4 oz.)	133	119	41
Grouper, cooked, dry heat (4 oz.)	134	60	27
Haddock, cooked, dry heat (4 oz.)	127	99	35
Herring, cooked, dry heat (4 oz.)	230	130	48
Mackerel, cooked, dry heat (4 oz.)	297	94	50
Mahi-Mahi, cooked, dry heat (4 oz.)	124	128	39
Monkfish, cooked, dry heat (4 oz.)	110	26	34
Orange roughy, cooked, dry heat (4 oz.)	101	92	51
Perch, cooked, dry heat (4 oz.)	133	90	27
Salmon, pink, cooked, dry heat (4 oz.)	169	98	39
Smelt, rainbow, cooked, dry heat (4 oz.)	141	87	40
Snapper, cooked, dry heat (4 oz.)	145	65	35
Sole, cooked, dry heat (4 oz.)	133	119	41
Swordfish, cooked, dry heat (4 oz.)	176	130	38
Tilapia, cooked, dry heat (4 oz.)	195	74	18
Trout, rainbow, farmed, cooked, dry heat (4 oz.)	192	48	33
Trout, rainbow, wild, cooked, dry heat (4 oz.)	170	64	36
Tuna, yellowfin, cooked, dry heat (4 oz.)	158	53	46

Food item Description/portion size	Calories	Sodium	ANDI score
Prepared (processed)			
Fish fillet, batter-coated, fried (4 oz.)	263	603	10
Fish sticks, frozen, heated (4 sticks)	305	652	12
Shellfish			
Clams, breaded, fried (4 oz.)	229	413	107
Clams, cooked, moist heat (4 oz.)	168	127	341
Clams, raw (4 oz.)	84	64	341
Crab, Alaska king, cooked, moist heat (4 oz.)	110	1216	97
Crab, blue, cooked, moist heat (4 oz.)	116	316	71
Crayfish, farmed, cooked, moist heat (4 oz.)	99	110	45
Lobster, cooked, moist heat (4 oz.)	111	431	43
Mussels, cooked, moist heat (4 oz.)	195	418	102
Oysters, farmed, raw (4 oz.)	67	202	292
Scallops, breaded, fried (6 scallops)	200	432	15
Scallops, steamed (4 oz.)	120	478	24
Shrimp, breaded, fried (4 oz.)	274	390	17
Shrimp, cooked, moist heat (4 oz.)	112	254	38
Squid, fried (4 oz.)	198	347	26
Squid, raw (4 oz.)	104	50	45

Frozen Foods

Breakfast			
French toast (2 slices)	251	584	22*
French toast sticks (4 slices)	411	399	10*
Waffle (2 waffles)	176	524	28*
Main Meal			
Chicken pot pie (217g)	484	857	7

* Artificially inflated nutrient score due to fortification with vitamins and minerals.

Food item Description/portion size	Calo ries	Sod ium	ANDI score
Pasta			
Cheese lasagna (240g)	298	660	26*
Healthy Choice Beef Macaroni (240g)	211	444	33*
Lasagna w/ meat & sauce (240g)	305	672	25*
Pizza			
Cheese pizza, regular crust (162g)	434	724	14*
Sausage & pepperoni pizza (146g)	385	854	12*
Vegetables			
French fried potatoes, frozen (14 fries)	140	21	11
Hashed brown potatoes, frozen (1-1/2 cups)	510	80	7
Onion rings, breaded (11 rings)	318	293	6
Potato puffs, frozen (1-1/2 cups)	426	1432	10

Fruit

	Calo ries	Sod ium	ANDI score
Apples			
Applesauce (1 cup)	194	8	31
Apple, dried (1/2 cup)	104	37	22
Apple, fresh (1 apple)	72	1	76
Apricots			
Apricots, dried, unsweetened (1/3 cup)	104	4	21
Apricots, fresh (4 apricots)	67	1	64
Avocado			
Avocado, fresh (half)	182	3	37
Banana			
Banana, fresh (1 banana)	105	1	30

Artificially inflated nutrient score due to fortification with vitamins and minerals.

Food item *Description/portion size*	Calo ries	Sod ium	ANDI score
Blackberries			
Blackberries, fresh (1-1/2 cups)	93	2	178
Blackberries, unsweetened, frozen (1-1/2 cups)	145	2	110
Blueberries			
Blueberries, canned in heavy syrup (1-1/2 cups)	338	12	8
Blueberries, fresh (1-1/2 cups)	123	2	130
Blueberries, frozen, sweetened (1-1/2 cups)	279	3	9
Blueberries, frozen, unsweetened (1-1/2 cups)	119	2	140
Cantaloupe			
Cantaloupe, fresh (1-1/2 cups)	82	38	100
Cherries			
Cherries, canned, in heavy syrup (1-1/2 cups)	315	11	9
Cherries, fresh (1-1/2 cups)	137	0	68
Cherries, sweetened, frozen (1-1/2 cups)	346	4	46
Cranberries			
Cranberries, fresh (1/2 cup)	25	1	234
Cranberry sauce, sweetened, canned (1/4 cup)	105	20	3
Currants			
Currants (1/4 cup)	102	3	21
Dates			
Dates, domestic (1/4 cup)	125	1	19
Dates, medjool (2 dates)	133	0	19
Figs			
Figs, dried (1/4 cup)	124	5	25
Figs, fresh (3 figs)	111	2	62

Food item Description/portion size	Calories	Sodium	ANDI score
Fruit Cocktail			
Fruit cocktail, canned in heavy syrup (1-1/2 cups)	272	22	8
Fruit cocktail, canned in juice (1-1/2 cups)	164	14	14
Fruit cocktail, canned in light syrup (1-1/2 cups)	207	22	11
Grapefruit			
Grapefruit, fresh (1-1/2 cups)	144	0	102
Grapes			
Grapes, fresh (1-1/2 cups)	92	3	31
Honeydew			
Honeydew, fresh (1-1/2 cups)	96	48	45
Kiwi			
Kiwi, fresh (2 kiwis)	93	5	97
Lemon			
Lemon, fresh (1 lemon)	22	3	280
Lemon, juice (1 tsp.)	1	0	141
Lime			
Lime, fresh (1 lime)	20	1	94
Lime, juice (1 tsp.)	1	0	99
Mango			
Mango, fresh (1 mango)	135	4	51
Nectarine			
Nectarine, fresh (1-1/2 cups)	91	0	41

Food item Description/portion size	Calories	Sodium	ANDI score
Oranges			
Orange, fresh (1 orange)	62	0	109
Orange, Mandarin, canned in juice (1-1/2 cups)	138	19	67
Orange, Mandarin, canned in light syrup (1-1/2 cups)	231	23	29
Papaya			
Papaya, fresh (1-1/2 cups)	82	6	118
Peaches			
Peaches, dried (1/4 cup)	96	3	24
Peaches, fresh (1 peach)	38	0	73
Peaches, halves, canned in heavy syrup (1-1/2 cups)	291	24	16
Peaches, halves, canned in light syrup (1-1/2 cups)	203	19	21
Peaches, halves, canned in own juice (1-1/2 cups)	164	15	29
Peaches, slices, frozen, sweetened (1-1/2 cups)	353	23	49
Pears			
Pears, canned, in heavy syrup (1-1/2 cups)	295	20	12
Pears, canned, in juice (1-1/2 cups)	186	15	19
Pears, canned, in light syrup (1-1/2 cups)	215	19	15
Pears, fresh (1 pear)	96	2	46
Pineapple			
Pineapple, canned, in heavy syrup (1-1/2 cups)	297	4	18
Pineapple, canned, in own juice (1-1/2 cups)	224	4	24
Pineapple, fresh (1-1/2 cups)	112	2	64
Plums			
Plums, fresh (1-1/2 cups)	114	0	157

Food item *Description/portion size*	*Calo ries*	*Sod ium*	*ANDI score*
Prunes			
Prunes, dried (1/4 cup)	102	1	47
Raisins			
Raisins (1/4 cup)	108	4	16
Raspberries			
Raspberries, fresh (1-1/2 cups)	96	2	145
Raspberries, sweetened, frozen (1-1/2 cups)	386	4	18
Strawberries			
Strawberries, fresh (1-1/2 cups)	69	2	212
Strawberries, frozen, sweetened (1-1/2 cups)	298	4	29
Strawberries, frozen, unsweetened (1-1/2 cups)	78	4	174
Tangerine			
Tangerine, fresh (2 tangerines)	89	3	72
Watermelon			
Watermelon, fresh (2.5 cups)	114	4	91

Food item Description/portion size	Calo ries	Sod ium	ANDI score

Meat

Beef

Beef, bottom round, 1/8" fat, braised (3 oz.)	210	37	21
Beef, chuck, pot roast, 1/8" fat, braised (3 oz.)	251	43	17
Beef, flank, separable lean only, 0" fat, broiled (4 oz.)	213	64	27
Beef, ground, 85% lean meat, broiled (4 oz.)	284	82	20
Beef, jerky (2 oz.)	232	1255	13
Beef, prime rib, 1/8" fat, roasted (4 oz.)	454	74	12
Beef, short loin, porterhouse, 1/4" fat, broiled (4 oz.)	388	69	12
Beef, tenderloin, 1/8" fat, broiled (3 oz.)	292	47	13
Beef, top round, London broil, 0" fat, broiled (4 oz.)	211	46	26
Corned beef brisket, cooked (4 oz.)	285	1286	16
Pastrami (3 oz.)	124	753	28

Cold Cuts

Bologna, beef & pork (2 slices)	175	417	13
Chicken roll, light meat (2 slices)	87	331	15
Ham, 11% fat (2 slices)	92	739	24
Salami, beef & pork (2 slices)	115	490	18
Turkey roll, light meat (2 slices)	83	277	23
Turkey, white, rotisserie, deli cut (2 oz.)	64	680	33

Hot Dogs & Sausage

Beef & pork chorizo (4 oz.)	516	1400	12
Bratwurst, beef & pork (4 oz.)	337	962	13
Hot dog, beef (1 hot dog)	148	513	8
Hot dog, pork (1 hot dog)	153	631	18
Hot dog, tofu (1 hot dog)	163	330	23
Hot dog, turkey (1 hot dog)	102	642	13
Italian sausage, pork (4 oz.)	390	1369	13
Italian sausage, turkey (4 oz.)	179	1052	35
Kielbasa, beef & pork (4 oz.)	352	1220	11

Food item *Description/portion size*	*Calo ries*	*Sod ium*	*ANDI score*
Knockwurst, beef & pork (4 oz.)	348	1055	9
Pepperoni, beef & pork (2 oz.)	264	1014	10
Smoked sausage, beef & pork (4 oz.)	363	1033	6

Lamb
Lamb, leg, separable lean & fat, 1/4" fat, roasted (3 oz.)	206	57	21
Lamb, loin chops, lean, 1/8" fat, broiled (4 oz.)	337	88	16
Lamb, ground (4 oz.)	321	92	18

Misc. Meat
Liver pâté (4 Tbsp.)	166	362	19
Liverwurst spread (1/4 cup)	168	385	42
Pork rinds, fried (2 oz.)	309	1042	5
Smoked meat stick (2 sticks)	218	586	7

Pork
Bacon (2 slices)	68	291	12
Bacon, Canadian (2 oz.)	89	799	28
Country Style Ribs, separable lean & fat, roasted (4 oz.)	372	59	17
Ground pork (4 oz.)	337	83	17
Ham, cured, boneless, 11% fat, roasted (4 oz.)	202	1701	26
Ham, cured, extra lean, 5% fat, roasted (4 oz.)	164	1364	30
Ham, honey, smoked (4 oz.)	138	1021	18
Pork chops, center cut, lean, panfried (4 oz.)	314	91	22
Pork chops, center cut, lean, broiled (4 oz.)	229	68	32
Pork loin, tenderloin, lean, roasted (4 oz.)	186	64	37
Pork loin, whole, separable lean & fat, roasted (4 oz.)	281	67	23

Poultry
Chicken, breast, meat only, roasted (4 oz.)	187	84	27
Chicken, drumstick, meat & skin, flour coated, fried (4 oz.)	278	101	14
Chicken, drumstick, meat only, roasted (4 oz.)	195	108	20

Food item *Description/portion size*	Calo ries	Sod ium	ANDI score
Chicken, liver (4 oz.)	189	86	138
Chicken, wing, meat & skin, flour coated, fried (4 oz.)	364	87	10
Chicken, wing, meat only, roasted (4 oz.)	230	104	18
Cornish game hen, meat only, roasted (4 oz.)	152	71	23
Duck, meat & skin, roasted (4 oz.)	382	67	10
Duck, meat only, roasted (4 oz.)	228	74	21
Turkey, bacon (0.44 oz.)	48	285	9
Turkey, fryer roaster, roasted (4 oz.)	159	64	28
Turkey, ground (4 oz.)	266	121	17

Nuts & Seeds

Nut Butter

Almond (2 Tbsp.)	203	4	20
Cashew (2 Tbsp.)	188	5	13
Peanut (2 Tbsp.)	188	147	18
Tahini (sesame butter) (2 Tbsp.)	178	34	32

Nuts

Almonds, blanched (1/4 cup)	211	10	25
Almonds, dry roasted, no salt (1/4 cup)	206	0	25
Almonds, dry roasted, salted (1/4 cup)	206	117	25
Brazil (1/4 cup)	230	1	116
Cashews, dry roasted, no salt (1/4 cup)	197	5	14
Cashews, raw (34.25g)	189	4	16
Cashews, salted (1/4 cup)	197	219	14
Hazelnuts (filberts) (1/4 cup)	212	0	29
Macadamia, dry roasted, no salt (1/4 cup)	241	1	9
Macadamia, dry roasted, salted (1/4 cup)	240	89	9
Macadamia, raw (1/4 cup)	241	2	10
Peanuts, all types, dry roasted, no salt (1/4 cup)	214	2	19

Food item Description/portion size	Calo ries	Sod ium	ANDI score
Peanuts, all types, dry roasted, salted (1/4 cup)	214	297	19
Peanuts, all types, oil roasted, salted (1/4 cup)	216	115	17
Pecans (1/4 cup)	187	0	34
Pine nuts (pignolia) (1 Tbsp.)	58	0	10
Pistachio, dry roasted, no salt (1/4 cup)	183	3	29
Pistachio, dry roasted, salted (1/4 cup)	182	130	29
Walnuts (1/4 cup)	196	1	29

Seeds

Flaxseed (2 Tbsp.)	118	8	44
Pumpkin (1/4 cup)	187	6	36
Sesame (2 Tbsp.)	102	2	41
Sunflower (1/4 cup)	186	1	45

Snacks

Bars, Non-Candy

Crisped rice bar w/ chocolate chips (1 bar)	115	79	16
Fabes Bar (1 bar)	230	5	26
Granola bar, almond, hard (1 bar)	117	60	9
Granola bar, chocolate chip, hard (1 bar)	103	81	11
Granola bar, chocolate chip, chocolate coated, soft (1 bar)	132	57	9
Granola bar, chocolate chip, soft (1 bar)	178	116	12
Granola bar, oats, fruits & nuts (1 bar)	95	60	22
Granola bar, peanut butter, chocolate coated, soft (1 bar)	187	71	8
Granola bar, peanut butter, hard (1 bar)	114	67	9
Granola bar, plain, hard (1 bar)	115	72	11
Granola bar, raisin, soft (1 bar)	127	80	11
Halvah bar (1/4 bar)	266	111	13
Health Valley Fat-Free Apple Bakes (1 bar)	70	30	22
Kashi Go Lean Peanut & Chocolate Bar (1 bar)	290	280	13
Kellogg's All Bran Breakfast Bar, Honey Oat (1 bar)	130	170	20

Food item Description/portion size	Calo ries	Sod ium	ANDI score
Kellogg's Nutri Grain Cereal Bar (1 bar) (37g)	136	110	30*
Kellogg's Pop Tarts, Brown Sugar Cinnamon (1 Pop Tart)	219	214	8*
Kellogg's Rice Krispies Treats Squares (1 bar) (1.13 oz.)	133	112	20*
Pop Tarts Toaster Pastry (1 pastry)	219	214	8*

Candy, Chocolate

3 Musketeers Bar(1 bar)	94	44	10
Dr. Fuhrman's Date Nut Pop 'Ems, chocolate (3 balls)	125	2	36
Kit Kat Wafer Bar (1 bar)	220	23	9
Kudos Whole Grain Bars, Chocolate Chip (1 bar) (1 oz.)	124	79	25*
M&M's Milk Chocolate Candies (about 60 pieces)	206	26	4
M&M's Peanut Chocolate Candies (about 24 pieces)	244	23	18
Milk chocolate bar w/ almonds (1 piece)	216	30	20
Milk chocolate candy bar (44g) (1 bar)	235	35	21
Milk chocolate coated raisins (1/4 cup) (45 pieces)	176	16	20
Milk chocolate covered peanuts (1/4 cup)	210	17	19
Milky Way Bar (1 bar)	228	129	12
Mounds Bar (1 bar)	262	78	7
Nestle Baby Ruth Bar (Fun Size Bar) (1 bar)	99	46	11
Nestle Butter Finger (Fun Size Bar) (1 bar)	100	45	11
Reese's Peanut Butter Cups (2 pieces)	175	107	13
Snickers Bar (1 bar)	265	129	14
Twix Caramel Cookie Bars (58g)	291	113	10

Candy, Non-Chocolate

Butterscotch candy (5 pieces)	117	117	0
Caramel candy (3 pieces)	116	74	4
Chewing gum, stick (1 stick)	7	0	1
Dr. Fuhrman's Date Nut Pop 'Ems, Cinnamon (3 balls)	125	2	31
Dr. Fuhrman's Date Nut Pop 'Ems, Plain (3 balls)	125	2	20
Gumdrops (8 gumdrops)	114	13	0
Jelly beans (10 jelly beans)	106	14	0

* Artificially inflated nutrient score due to fortification with vitamins and minerals.

Food item *Description / portion size*	*Calo ries*	*Sod ium*	*ANDI score*
Marshmallows (4 marshmallows)	92	23	0
Nougat candy (2 pieces)	111	9	4
Peanut brittle (1.25 oz.)	172	158	5
Sesame crunch candy (17 pieces)	154	50	16
Skittles Original Bite Size Candies (30 pieces)	130	5	7
Starburst Fruit Chews (6 pieces)	119	17	6
Taffy (2 pieces)	113	27	0
Toffee (1 piece)	214	127	2
Tootsie Roll Chocolate Flavor Roll (5 pieces)	128	15	2

Cookies

Animal crackers (12 crackers)	134	118	8*
Arrowroot cookies (12 cookies)	134	118	8*
Barbara's Bakery Fat-Free Oatmeal Raisin Mini Cookies (6)	110	105	9*
Butter cookies, ready to eat (6 cookies)	140	105	7*
Chocolate chip cookies (3 cookies)	147	89	7*
Chocolate chip cookies, lower-fat (3 cookies)	136	113	7*
Chocolate coated Graham crackers (2 cookies)	136	81	10*
Chocolate covered marshmallow cookies (2 cookies)	109	44	5*
Chocolate sandwich cookies w/ creme filling (3 cookies)	140	145	9*
Chocolate sandwich cookies w/ extra creme filling (2)	129	91	7
Fig bars (2 bars)	111	112	8*
Frookie Apple Cinnamon Oat Bran Cookies (2 cookies)	90	80	12
Fudge cake cookies (1 cookies)	73	40	7*
Ginger snaps (4 cookies)	116	183	9*
Health Valley Fat-Free Original Healthy Chip Cookies (3)	100	90	9*
Health Valley Fat-Free Raisin Oatmeal Cookies (3)	100	80	9*
Health Valley Fat-Free Raspberry Center Cookies (1 cookie)	70	20	13*
Nabisco Snackwell's Caramel Delights Cookies (36g)	138	66	3*
Nabisco Snackwell's Devil's Food Cookie Cakes (32g)	98	56	5*
Oatmeal cookies w/ raisins, ready to eat (2 cookies)	162	138	7*
Oatmeal cookies without raisins (2 cookies)	134	179	6*

* Artificially inflated nutrient score due to fortification with vitamins and minerals.

Food item Description/portion size	Calo ries	Sod ium	ANDI score
Peanut butter cookie, ready to eat (2 cookies)	143	124	7*
Peanut butter sandwich cookie, ready to eat (2 cookies)	134	103	8*
Pecan shortbread cookie, ready to eat (2 cookies)	152	79	5*
Shortbread cookie, ready to eat (4 cookies)	161	146	7*
Sugar cookie, ready to eat (2 cookies)	143	107	5*
Sugar wafer cookie w/ creme filling (8 cookies)	143	41	4*
Vanilla sandwich cookie w/ creme filling (3 cookies)	145	105	6*
Vanilla wafer cookie (5 cookies)	142	92	6*

Doughnuts

Chocolate coated cake doughnut (1 doughnut)	204	184	6
Doughnut w/ creme filling (1 doughnut)	307	263	8
Doughnut w/ jelly filling (1 doughnut)	289	249	6
Glazed cake doughnut (1 doughnut)	192	181	5
Glazed French cruller (1 cruller)	169	141	5

Fruit Snacks

Banana chips (1-1/2 oz.)	221	3	8
Betty Crocker Fruit by the Foot (1 strip)	80	50	8*
Betty Crocker Fruit Gushers (.9 oz pouch)	90	55	7*
Betty Crocker Fruit Roll Ups (1 Roll Up)	50	55	12*
Betty Crocker Fruit Roll Ups w/ vitamin C (2 Roll Ups)	104	89	14*
Fruit leather roll (1 roll)	78	67	17

Gelatin & Pudding

Chocolate pudding mix, prepared w/ 2% milk (1 cup)	309	835	11
Chocolate pudding, fat-free (1 cup) (294g)	285	500	12
Gelatin mix, prepared w/ water (1 cup)	167	203	1
Rice pudding, prepared w/ 2% milk (1 cup)	320	314	10
Tapioca pudding, prepared w/ 2% milk (1 cup)	296	341	9
Vanilla pudding, prepared w/ 2% milk (1 cup)	283	445	10
Vanilla pudding, fat-free (1 cup) (280g)	260	596	8

* Artificially inflated nutrient score due to fortification with vitamins and minerals.

Food item Description/portion size	Calo ries	Sod ium	ANDI score
Chips			
Corn chips, plain (1 oz.)	153	179	6
Potato chips, barbecue (1 oz.)	139	213	13
Potato chips, fat-free, salted (1 oz.)	107	182	17
Potato chips, salted (1 oz.)	152	168	11
Potato chips, sour cream & onion flavor (1 oz.)	151	177	12
Potato chips, unsalted (1 oz.)	152	2	11
Tortilla chips, low-fat, baked w/ no fat (1 oz.)	118	119	9
Tortilla chips, nacho (1 oz.)	141	201	7
Tortilla chips, plain (1 oz.)	142	150	8
Tortilla chips, unsalted (1 oz.) (16 chips)	149	70	7
Tortilla chips, light, baked w/ less oil (1 oz.) (18 chips)	134	289	9
Miscellaneous Snacks			
Brown rice cakes (2 cakes)	70	59	12
Corn nuts (1 oz.)	126	156	8
Corn puffs, cheese flavored (1 oz.)	157	298	8
Popcorn cakes (2 items)	77	58	12
Quaker Plain Rice Cakes, salted (2 cakes)	70	30	11*
Popcorn			
Popcorn, air popped, no salt (4 cups) (4 cups)	122	1	16
Popcorn, oil popped, no salt (4 cups) (44g)	229	1	8
Pretzels			
Pretzels, chocolate-covered (5 pretzels)	252	313	4*
Pretzels, hard, salted (60g) (10 pretzels)	229	1029	13*
Pretzels, hard, unsalted (60g) (10 pretzels)	229	173	13*
Pretzels, soft (1 pretzel)	389	1615	11*
Pretzels, whole wheat (60g) (10 pretzels)	217	122	12

Artificially inflated nutrient score due to fortification with vitamins and minerals.

Soups & Stews

(all condensed soups; all prepared with water)

Beans, Peas, & Lentils

	Calories	Sodium	ANDI score
Black bean, condensed, canned (2 cups)	232	2396	36
Health Valley No Salt Added Organic Black Bean (2 cups)	260	50	90
Health Valley Fat-Free Black Bean & Vegetable (2 cups)	240	780	94
Health Valley Fat-Free Lentil & Carrot (2 cups)	220	900	97
Green pea, condensed, canned (2 cups)	330	1835	32

Beef, Chicken, & Seafood

	Calories	Sodium	ANDI score
Beef broth of bouillon, canned (2 cups)	34	1565	37
Beef broth of bouillon, powder (1 cube)	14	1019	15
Beef flavor Ramen noodle, dehydrated (43g)	187	861	14
Beef mushroom, condensed, canned (2 cups)	146	1884	18
Beef noodle, condensed, canned (2 cups)	166	1903	40
Vegetable beef, condensed, canned (2 cups)	156	1581	34
Chicken broth, cube (1 cube)	10	1152	20
Chicken broth, canned (2 cups)	78	1552	22
Campbell's Healthy Request Chicken Broth (2 cups)	34	771	70
Chicken-flavor Ramen noodle (43g)	188	891	10
Chicken gumbo, condensed (2 cups)	112	1908	41
Chicken noodle, condensed, canned (2 cups)	149	2212	18
Chicken vegetable, condensed, canned (2 cups)	149	1889	29
Cream of chicken, condensed, canned (2 cups)	234	1972	10
Campbell's Healthy Request Cream of Chicken (2 cups)	263	1619	12
Clam chowder, Manhattan, condensed, canned (2 cups)	156	1157	67
Clam chowder, New England, condensed, canned (2 cups)	190	1830	50

Vegetables

	Calories	Sodium	ANDI score
Imagine Creamy Butternut Squash (2 cups)	240	740	83
Cream of celery, condensed, canned (2 cups)	181	1898	11

Food item *Description/portion size*	*Calo ries*	*Sod ium*	*ANDI score*
Gazpacho, canned, ready to eat (2 cups)	93	1479	67
Minestrone, condensed, canned (2 cups)	164	1822	85
Cream of mushroom, condensed, canned (2 cups)	259	1762	8
Mushroom barley, condensed, canned (2 cups)	146	1781	29
Onion, condensed, canned (2 cups)	116	2106	16
Tomato, condensed, canned (2 cups)	171	1391	110
Health Valley No Salt Added Organic Tomato (2 cups)	160	70	96
Imagine Organic Creamy Tomato (2 cups)	180	1040	93
Vegetable broth, canned (2 cups)	30	1880	25
Vegetarian vegetable, condensed, canned (2 cups)	145	1644	68
Campbell's Healthy Request Vegetable (2 cups)	200	720	86
Health Valley No Salt Added Organic Vegetable (2 cups)	160	80	90
Healthy Choice Country Vegetable (2 cups)	200	960	89
Health Valley Fat-Free 14 Garden Vegetable (2 cups)	160	780	97
Imagine Low Sodium Vegetable Broth (2 cups)	40	280	40
Imagine Organic Vegetable Broth (2 cups)	60	920	40
Progresso Healthy Classics Vegetable (2 cups)	241	846	88
Westbrae Natural Fat-Free Santa Fe Vegetable (2 cups)	320	760	89

Soy Products

Soybean Products

Fermented soybean paste (miso) (2 Tbsp.)	68	1282	15
Soybean curd cheese (1/2 cup)	170	22	27
Soy burgers (1burger)	125	385	45

Tofu Products

Tofu (4 oz.)	69	9	86
Tofu hot dog (1 hot dog)	163	330	23
Tofu yogurt (1 cup)	246	92	17

Syrups, Sweeteners, Baking Items

Cocoa

Description	Calories	Sodium	ANDI score
Cocoa, unsweetened, dry (1 Tbsp.)	12	1	518

Chocolate Syrup

Description	Calories	Sodium	ANDI score
Chocolate syrup (2 Tbsp.)	105	27	5

Coconut

Description	Calories	Sodium	ANDI score
Coconut flakes, sweetened (1/4 cup)	88	47	5
Coconut milk (8 fluid oz.)	552	36	7
Coconut water (8 fluid oz.)	46	252	38

Frosting

Description	Calories	Sodium	ANDI score
Chocolate frosting, ready to eat (38g)	151	70	2
Vanilla frosting, ready to eat (38g)	160	70	3

Pie Crust

Description	Calories	Sodium	ANDI score
Pie crust, prepared, baked (1 slice)	121	125	7*

Sweeteners

Description	Calories	Sodium	ANDI score
Brown sugar (1 tsp.)	11	1	2
Corn syrup (2 Tbsp.)	128	28	1
Honey (1 Tbsp.)	64	1	1
Molasses (1 Tbsp.)	58	7	15
Molasses, blackstrap (1 Tbsp.)	47	11	33
White granulated sugar (1 tsp.)	15	0	0

Syrups

Description	Calories	Sodium	ANDI score
Chocolate syrup (2 Tbsp.)	105	27	5
Maple syrup (1/4 cup)	209	7	4

* Artificially inflated nutrient score due to fortification with vitamins and minerals.

Food item Description/portion size	Calo ries	Sod ium	ANDI score
Pancake syrup (1/4 cup)	187	66	1
Pancake syrup, reduced-calorie (1/4 cup)	98	120	0

Vegetables

Alfalfa sprouts (1 cup)	10	2	130
Artichoke, boiled, drained (1 artichoke)	60	114	244
Arugula (5 cups)	25	27	559
Asparagus, cooked (1-1/2 cups)	59	38	234
Bamboo shoots, canned (1 cup)	25	9	144
Bean sprouts (1 cup)	53	11	444
Beets, boiled (1-1/2 cups)	112	196	97
Bok choy (1-1/2 cups)	31	87	824
Broccoli, boiled (1-1/2 cups)	82	96	342
Broccoli, uncooked (1-1/2 cups)	45	44	376
Brussels sprouts, boiled (1-1/2 cups)	84	49	672
Cabbage, boiled (1-1/2 cups)	50	18	481
Cabbage, raw (1-1/2 cups)	32	24	420
Cabbage, red, cooked (1-1/2 cups)	65	18	330
Cabbage, red, raw (1-1/2 cups)	33	28	352
Cabbage, savoy, raw (1-1/2 cups)	28	29	374
Carrots, boiled (1/2 cup)	27	45	336
Carrots, raw (1-1/2 cups)	75	126	240
Cauliflower, boiled (1-1/2 cups)	43	28	295
Cauliflower, raw (1-1/2 cups)	38	45	285
Celery (2 stalks)	11	64	135
Chicory greens, uncooked (1-1/2 cups)	62	122	591
Chili peppers, green, hot (1 item)	18	3	323
Chinese or Napa cabbage, cooked (1-1/2 cups)	20	18	704
Chinese or Napa cabbage, raw (1-1/2 cups)	18	10	600
Collard greens, boiled (1-1/2 cups)	74	46	1000

Food item Description/portion size	Calo ries	Sod ium	ANDI score
Corn, sweet, white, boiled (1-1/2 cups)	266	42	25
Cucumber (1 cucumber)	45	6	50
Dandelion greens, boiled (1-1/2 cups)	52	69	329
Eggplant, cooked (1-1/2 cups)	50	1	149
Escarole (3 cups)	25	33	322
Garlic clove (1 clove)	4	1	58
Green beans, boiled (2 cups)	87	2	74
Green peas (1-1/2 cups)	202	7	70
Jalapeno peppers (1/8 cup)	7	0	164
Kale, boiled (1-1/2 cups)	55	45	1000
Kale, uncooked (1-1/2 cups)	50	43	905
Kohlrabi (1-1/2 cups)	54	40	393
Leeks (2 cups)	109	36	80
Lettuce, iceberg (5 cups)	38	28	110
Lettuce, romaine (5 cups)	48	22	389
Mushrooms (1-1/2 cups)	23	4	135
Mushrooms, boiled (1-1/2 cups)	66	5	119
Mushrooms, shitake, cooked (1-1/2 cups)	120	9	55
Mustard greens, boiled (1-1/2 cups)	32	34	1000
Okra, boiled (1-1/2 cups)	53	14	139
Olives, black, canned (3 olives)	15	115	17
Onions, boiled (1/3 cup)	31	2	50
Onions, raw (1/2 cup)	34	2	47
Parsley (1 Tbsp.)	1	2	480
Parsnips (1-1/2 cups)	166	23	37
Peppers, green (or sweet), cooked (1-1/2 cups)	57	4	181
Peppers, green (or sweet), raw (1-1/2 cups)	45	7	258
Pepper, red (sweet) (1-1/2 cups)	58	4	420
Potato, red, flesh & skin (184g)	132	11	43
Potatoes, flesh & skin (1 potato)	142	11	43
Potatoes, flesh only, baked (1-1/2 cups)	170	9	31
Potatoes, mashed, prepared w/milk & butter (1-1/2 cups)	306	517	16

Food item Description/portion size	Calories	Sodium	ANDI score
Pumpkin, canned (1/2 cup)	42	6	372
Radicchio (2 cups)	18	18	359
Radish (6 radishes)	4	11	554
Rhubarb (1 cup)	25	5	106
Sauerkraut, canned (1/8 cup)	6	195	98
Scallions (1 Tbsp.)	2	0	173
Snow or sugar peas (1-1/2 cups)	40	4	127
Snow or sugar peas, boiled (1-1/2 cups)	101	10	113
Spinach, boiled (1-1/2 cups)	62	189	697
Spinach, uncooked (5 cups)	34	118	739
Squash, acorn (winter), boiled (1-1/2 cups)	125	11	60
Squash, butternut (winter), baked (1-1/2 cups)	122	12	159
Squash (summer) (2 cups)	72	4	141
Squash, spaghetti (winter) (1-1/2 cups)	63	42	52
Squash (winter), all varieties, baked (1-1/2 cups)	113	3	137
String beans, boiled (1-1/2 cups)	65	6	75
Sweet potato (1-1/2 cups)	378	134	83
Swiss chard, boiled (1-1/2 cups)	52	470	670
Tomatillo (2 tomatillos)	22	1	72
Tomato, cooked (1 cup)	43	26	190
Tomato, paste, (2 Tbsp.)	27	259	197
Tomato, paste, no salt (2 Tbsp.)	27	32	197
Tomato, uncooked (1 item)	22	6	164
Tomato, sun-dried (1/2 cup)	70	566	113
Tomato, whole, canned (1 cup)	41	307	163
Tomato, whole, canned, no salt added (1 cup)	46	24	163
Turnip greens, boiled (1-1/2 cups)	43	63	1000
Turnips (1 turnip)	34	82	337
Water chestnuts (1 cup)	70	11	19
Watercress (3 cups)	11	42	1000
Yams (1-1/2 cups)	266	20	23
Zucchini (2-1/2 cups)	45	28	222

References

1. Tucker KL; Hallfrisch J; Qiao N; et al. "The combination of high fruit and vegetable and low saturated fat intakes is more protective against mortality in aging men than is either alone: the Baltimore Longitudinal Study of Aging." *J Nutr* 2005;135(3):556-61.

2. Esselstyn CB. "Updating a 12-year experience with arrest and reversal therapy for coronary heart disease (an overdue requiem for palliative cardiology)." *Am J Cardiol* 1999;84(3):339-41.

3. Bazzano LA; He J; Ogden LG; et al. "Fruit and vegetable intake and risk of cardiovascular disease in US adults: the first National Health and Nutrition Examination Survey Epidemiologic Follow-up Study." *Am J Clin Nutr* 2002;76(1):93-9.

   Dauchet L; Amouyel P; Hercberg S; Dallongeville J. "Fruit and vegetable consumption and risk of coronary heart disease: a meta-analysis of cohort studies." *J Nutr* 2006;136(10):2588-93.

   Genkinger JM; Platz EA; Hoffman SC; et al. "Fruit, vegetable, and antioxidant intake and all-cause, cancer, and cardiovascular disease mortality in a community-dwelling population in Washington County, Maryland." *Am J Epidemiol* 2004;160(12): 1223-33.

   Sauvaget C; Nagano J; Allen N; Kodama K. "Vegetable and fruit intake and stroke mortality in the Hiroshima/Nagasaki Life Span Study." *Stroke* 2003;34(10):2355-60.

Rissanen TH; Voutilainen S; Virtanen JK; et al. "Low intake of fruits, berries and vegetables is associated with excess mortality in men: the Kuopio Ischaemic Heart Disease Risk Factor (KIHD) Study." *J Nutr* 2003;133(1):199-204.

Joffe M; Robertson A. "The potential contribution of increased vegetable and fruit consumption to health gain in the European Union." *Public Health Nutr* 2001;4(4):893-901.

Tobias M; Turley M; Stefanogiannis N; et al. "Vegetable and fruit intake and mortality from chronic disease in New Zealand." *Aust N Z J Public Health* 2006;30(1):26-31.

Michels KB; Wolk A. "A prospective study of variety of healthy foods and mortality in women." *Int J Epidemiol* 2002;31(4):847-54.

Martin A; Cherubini A; Andres-Lacueva C; et al. "Effects of fruits and vegetables on levels of vitamins E and C in the brain and their association with cognitive performance." *J Nutr Health Aging* 2002;6(6):392-404.

Liu RH. "Health benefits of fruits and vegetables are from additive and synergistic combinations of phytochemicals." *Am J Clin Nutr* 2003:78(3Suppl):517S-520S.

4. Roth GS; Ingram DK; Black A; Lane MA. "Effects of reduced energy intake on the biology of aging: the primate model." *Eur J Clin Nutr* 2000;54 Suppl 3:S15-20.

5. Kelemen LE; Kushi LH; Jacobs DR; Cerhan JR. "Associations of dietary protein with disease and mortality in a prospective study of postmenopausal women." *Am J Epidemiol* 2005;161(3):239-49.

6. Rose W. "The amino acid requirements of adult man." *Nutritional Abstracts and Reviews* 1957;27:631.

7. Kelemen LE; Kushi LH; Jacobs DR; Cerhan JR. "Associations of dietary protein with disease and mortality in a prospective study

of postmenopausal women." *Am J Epidemiol* 2005;161(3):239-49.

Kant AK; Schatzkin A; Graubard BI; Schairer C. "A prospective study of diet quality and mortality in women." *JAMA* 2000;283(16):2109-15.

Meydani M. "Nutrition interventions in aging and age-associated disease." *Ann N Y Acad Sci* 2001;928:226-35.

8. Hardage M. "Nutritional studies of vegetarians." *Journal of the American Dietetic Association* 1966;48:25.

9. Jenkins DJ; Kendall CW; Popovich DG; et al. "Effects of a very-high-fiber vegetable, fruit and nut diet on serum lipids and colonic function." *Metabolism* 2001:50(4);494-503.

10. Forman D; Bulwer BE. "Cardiovascular disease: optimal approaches to risk factor modification of diet and lifestyle." *Curr Treat Options Cardiovasc Med* 2006;8(1):47-57.

    Bazzano LA; Serdula MK; Liu S. "Dietary intake of fruits and vegetables and risk of cardiovascular disease." *Curr Atheroscler Rep* 2003;5(6):492-9.

11. Mai V; Kant AK; Flood A; et al. "Diet quality and subsequent cancer incidence and mortality in a prospective cohort of women." *Int J Epidemiol* 2005;34(1):54-60.

    Martínez ME. "Primary prevention of colorectal cancer: lifestyle, nutrition, exercise." *Recent Results Cancer Res* 2005;166:177-211.

    Giovannucci E. "Modifiable risk factors for colon cancer." *Gastroenterol Clin North Am* 2002;31(4):925-43.

Eat Right America

O ur mission is to make essential nutritional information available to people everywhere. We hope your interest will be sparked through this guide, and that you will begin the exhilarating journey towards optimal health, vitality, longevity, ideal weight, and freedom from the grip of chronic and devastating diseases. For complete information, we urge you to get the comprehensive two-book set, *Eat For Health*. The total *Eat For Health* program provides you with a deep reservoir of knowledge and a wealth of delicious, high-nutrient recipes that will help ensure that you achieve your optimal weight and reclaim your health.

We are prepared to help you with the tools you need to achieve your health goals, and we look forward to guiding you and being a vital part of your support community on your exciting journey.

Please visit us at our website www.EatRightAmerica.com or call (877) ERA-4-USA.

About the Author

Joel Fuhrman, M.D., is a board-certified family physician specializing in lifestyle and nutritional medicine in Flemington, New Jersey, and a graduate of the University of Pennsylvania School of Medicine.

As one of the country's leading experts on nutritional and natural healing, Dr. Fuhrman has been featured in hundreds of magazines and on major radio and television shows, including: "Good Morning America," CNN, "Good Day NY," TV Food Network, and the Discovery Channel's "Second Opinion with Dr. Oz."

Dr. Fuhrman's recommendations are designed for people who desire superior health, effective weight control, and to reverse and prevent disease. His most recent books include *Eat to Live—The Revolutionary Formula for Fast and Sustained Weight Loss, Cholesterol Protection for Life, Disease-Proof Your Child—Feeding Kids Right,* and *Eat For Health.*

www.EatRightAmerica.com
(877) ERA-4-USA